MATHIAS MALZIEU

Diary
of a
Vampire
in
Pyjamas

Translated from the French by
Sam Alexander

Quercus

First published in Great Britain in 2016 by

Quercus Editions Ltd
Carmelite House
50 Victoria Embankment
London EC4Y 0DZ

An Hachette UK company

A CIP catalogue record for this book is available
from the British Library

HB ISBN 978 1 78648 034 7
TPB ISBN 978 1 78648 035 4
EBOOK ISBN 978 1 78648 037 8

Every effort has been made to contact copyright holders.
However, the publishers will be glad to rectify in future editions
any inadvertent omissions brought to their attention.

'Jubilee Street', by Nick Cave and Warren Ellis (lyrics by Nick Cave),
reproduced by kind permission of Mute Song Limited.

10 9 8 7 6 5 4 3 2

Text designed and typeset by CC Book Production.
Printed and bound in Great Britain by Clays Ltd, St Ives Plc.

For Rosy – *ma fleur de combat* –
my sister, my father and all those
who didn't jump ship in the storm

Speed on, my Book! spread your white sails, my
    little bark, athwart the imperious waves!
Chant on – sail on – bear o'er the boundless blue,
    from me, to every shore,
This song for mariners and all their ships.

Walt Whitman
from 'In Cabin'd Ships at Sea'

It was the first time a patient had come to see me on
a skateboard, that's for sure.

Professor Peffault de Latour

I've just hitchhiked across hell. Real hell. Not the one with fires burning everywhere and men with horns listening to heavy metal. No, the one where you think: is my life over?

Messing about creatively:
a great way to make a living

6 November 2013

'You do too many things at once, you're not twenty any more,' people would say to me.

I'll have a rest when I'm dead.

I'm an adrenaline junkie. I've got Ali Baba's cave for brains, crammed so full my eye sockets could burst. I'm never bored, unless people slow me down. There's a firecracker in my heart and lava flowing in my veins. I'm always on the lookout for the electric spasm of surprise. I don't know how else to live.

I've always dreamed of being a superhero. To save myself, more than anything. But annihilating my demons would be too easy: the truth is I need them. Kill them and I kill myself. I've done my damnedest to be an inventor, a crooner, a semi-poet, an illusionist, a fake skater, a wild-animal impersonator and a devourer of women with skin like freshly tossed pancakes; now I'm an insomniac, anxious and exhausted from believing it all. Like I was taking the piss . . . out of myself.

My creative bulimia reached new heights when I lost my

mother. And it hasn't stopped rising. We all have crutches to lean on; mine are spinning tops. The rules are simple: don't stop, apply the brakes sparingly and, above all, don't allow yourself to be confined – literally or figuratively. Messing about creatively is a great way to earn a living.

Rock 'n' roll is an oasis of adrenaline for lost children. Imagine there's a 40,000-kilometre road going right around the world following the equator: my band Dionysos has driven it four times over in a van. We're an electric tribe formed by friends over twenty years ago. Being on stage makes my brain grow wings. Add friction to combustible emotions and I'm away. When I feel the hubbub of the crowd vibrating deep in my bones, I just have to give myself over to it. The trouble is, I give more than I've got. I'm a very stupid dragon who breathes fire and burns his own wings.

But on the horizon, I can just make out a desire for gentler things. Go down to the south of France for a bit, see my family somewhere other than in my dressing room after a gig, cycle to the cinema, maybe even become a dad.

Recently everything has concertinaed. I'm being whisked along by this tour/film/book rollercoaster,* so I assume my crushing tiredness is fairly standard. No holiday for two years, not much sleep, not much sun, but plenty of frenzied joy. Whatever it takes, I've got to finish this long sprint and reach the magical finishing line: the release of my first feature film. Can't fuck up a lucky break like that. This dream of

---

* I turned my novel *The Boy with the Cuckoo-Clock Heart* into a film entitled *Jack and the Cuckoo-Clock Heart.*

mine is six years in the making: now is not the time to crack. No slowing down!

It's the home straight: we're filming the music video for the Dionysos single 'Jack and the Cuckoo-Clock Heart', to be released alongside the animated film of the same title. Having left Paris in the small hours of the morning under washed-out stars, the band arrives at the film studio half-asleep. Early starts and rock 'n' roll go together about as well as a bowl of muesli and a glass of whisky. Everyone's talking at half speed. I've got bags under my eyes the size of ET's. Thanks to make-up, and the fact we're shooting in black and white, not everyone notices I'm actually 150 years old. I've rarely felt this tired before, but I'm wearing my trademark tight-fit suit and my pointy shoes. What could possibly go wrong?

The cameras and lights are in place, filming begins. We're pretending to play the song. Twisting this way and that. It's hard work and joyous, like jumping waves.

But at the end of each take, I feel like my heart is going to explode. The sensation of having a nut where my lungs should be and breathing through a blocked straw. Each jump costs me a fortune in breath. My head is spinning. My muscles are rigid. But they keep insisting on 'one more take'. I've done myself in on the long shots and we haven't even started the close-ups yet. I don't say anything, try to get my breath back during the breaks. The band is here, so are the people from the record label and the film. There's no going back, no slackening even. I have to do it all at full throttle. Inventing true stories makes me profoundly happy. Living them and sharing them, happier still. I try and concentrate on that.

Thirtieth take: I grit my teeth, try to conserve energy on the more extreme movements while keeping up the intensity. I feel seasick. No one notices, which is reassuring but only reinforces my sense of isolation.

The day is over at last. Everyone's happy. I catch sight of my reflection in the toilet mirror: I'm paler than Dracula. I don't say anything to anyone. But the next morning, I go for a blood test.

Necessary for life

I walk into one of those medical centres on the street, a sort of mini-hospital. An analysis lab, they call it. After a dose of empty silence, a jab in the arm and a biscuit, I'm free to go. 'You're very, very pale, Monsieur Malzieu . . . Will you be all right?' The nurse who has just given me the injection has the overtrained smile of compassion that's liable to freak you out.

It's the Friday before the Armistice bank holiday, so I won't get the results until Tuesday. I walk back up Boulevard Beaumarchais in slow motion. A little old lady, accompanied by a miniature dog with the same hairstyle as its owner, overtakes me on Place de la République. I buy a copy of *L'Équipe* and eat some chicken nuggets to avoid thinking about anything for several minutes at a stretch. It sort of works.

I get home. It's only round the corner but it's taken me a while. I'm stiff with cold inside my overcoat, though other people are strolling about in jumpers. I stopped taking the stairs weeks ago; today I'm even out of breath in the lift.

For months now, people have been telling me I'm very pale.

5

It's true I look like a vampire. It's no big deal though. I've been more tired than this on tour before. I lie down for a few minutes listening to Leonard Cohen and feel slightly better.

I call the taxi that's supposed to be taking me to the music-video edit. While I'm waiting, the telephone rings; a number I don't recognize.

'Hello. Monsieur Malzieu?'

'Yes.'

'Doctor Gelperowic here. The lab has just called to give me your results as a matter of urgency.'

'Really? They told me I wouldn't hear till Tuesday.'

'They decided to check your haemoglobin straight away and it's very low indeed. You're severely anaemic. Normal red blood cell levels are between 14 and 17 milligrams. Yours is 4.6. You need an immediate blood transfusion.'

'Sorry, what?'

'There isn't enough oxygen in your blood. You need to go to Accident and Emergency right now.'

'Right now?'

'With a red cell count that low, you shouldn't even be able to stand up . . . Avoid any physical exertion – you run the risk of having a heart attack.'

'Which hospital should I call?'

'The closest. And don't delay.'

Each sentence is a slap in the face. I'm knocked sideways.

I sit on my bed and try to get my emotions into some sort of order. My thoughts are blurry around the edges. Questions catapult back and forth, but not many answers. I play back the memory of the previous day, see myself bouncing around like a stupid dragon. I could have frazzled my heart live on film.

The telephone rings, the same number.

'It's Doctor Gelperowic again. We've just been given some new results.'

'And?'

'Unfortunately all three blood categories are affected. Your platelets are very low.'

'Platelets? I can't really remember . . .'

'They're the cells that prevent bleeding. You have very few.'

'What do you mean "very few"?'

'Normal is between 150,000 and 450,000 but you have 11,500. Under 20,000 and it's an automatic transfusion. Have you had any nosebleeds recently?'

'Yes.'

'Whatever you do, don't shave, don't handle sharp objects and try not to bang your head – we need to reduce the risk of haemorrhage. Your white blood cells are also affected, Monsieur Malzieu.'

'That's the immune system, right?'

'Yes. You have 750 neutrophils, when you should have double that. I won't disguise the fact that this is cause for concern.'

'Will the transfusion deal with that too?'

'Those cells can't be transfused. Until you get treatment, wash your hands as often as possible.'

'But what does it all mean?'

'You'll need to have further tests to get a diagnosis. They'll want to have a look at your bone marrow to see why your bloods are down.'

My heart is racing. My little apartment seems huge suddenly.

Haemoglobin, platelets, neutrophils, transfusion . . . The words crowd in like menacing shadows under my skull. I type bone marrow into the internet: '. . . plays a vital role in the working of the human body. It is responsible for the formation of particular cells (red and white blood cells and platelets), which are known as haematopoietic stem cells. Bone marrow cells produce the combination of blood cells that are necessary for life.'

Necessary for life?

Duty freaks

8 November 2013

8.30am. I arrive at the A&E department of Hôpital Cochin, as recommended by a doctor friend. The waiting room is a no-man's-land, separating the outside world from a sliding door disgorging armies of white coats. The place looks like the duty-free area in an airport after a plane crash.

On a noticeboard are written three rules (they're considerably less cool than the Three Rules in *Gremlins**):

3. For a non-urgent examination you will probably have to wait (several hours).
2. If your condition is serious, you will be treated quickly (less than half an hour).
1. If your condition is life-threatening, you will be treated immediately.

---

* In the 1980s fantasy film there are three rules for looking after a Mogwai: no bright light, don't get him wet, and never feed him after midnight, no matter how much he begs.

Two nurses escort me through the sliding door; I'm to be treated immediately. Everyone is very calm and, from the moment I hand over my blood test results, very quick. Questions, jabs, questions, a drip, a strange patch stuck on my sternum. Questions. Waiting.

Around me, it's the Court of Miracles. A man with a third knee high on his upper tibia, a woman with such a realistic black eye you'd swear it was movie make-up, an old lady repeating over and over again, 'Aaaah, it huuuuurts, they've amputated it,' even though all her arms and legs are sticking out, intact, from under her blanket. I'm sitting on my bed-on-wheels, a fat bit of sticky tape clinging to the hairs on my forearm. I look at the clock. The minute hand is moving at the speed of the hour hand. The batteries must have had it.

Two porters arrive and offer to help me into a wheelchair.

'But I can walk . . .'

'We've been told to transfer you in a chair, Monsieur.'

They bundle me up in blankets: let the karting commence! There's something Chaplinesque about whizzing along in a wheelchair in the sleet to the anxious click-clack of your beloved's high heels as she runs to keep up. I watch her losing ground, like a doe that's lost her way and is learning to gambol on tarmac. The clouds drift quickly between the buildings, sped on by the wind. My blanket slips off. The porters stop, pick it up and tuck me in like an elderly baby.

Eventually, we arrive at the entrance of the Achard building. An automatic door slowly opens. For a minute I think it's rain-ing inside the reception area, the atmosphere is that sad. The lift is reserved for people who are 'unwell'. That's not a lift I'd take ordinarily; it can't apply to me, surely. The corridors roll on by. My fear grows with every metre.

We reach a department marked Intensive Care. Everyone's wearing masks, white coats and potato-bag hairnets. It's reminiscent of a sci-fi nuclear power station. We're nearing the reactor: the sterile room. To gain access there's a freezer door leading to an airlock. There's medical equipment on a table and a sort of chimney, like a kitchen smoke-extractor. Surgeons' costumes are hanging on pegs. A light turns from red to green and a second door opens. With a gentle push, I'm wheeled inside. Blue walls and silence, broken by noises from the machines. What the hell am I doing here? The worst memory of my life comes back to me. When I lost my mum in a room just like this one. My heart is trying to climb out of my throat. The door closes, I'm trapped. Right now, I should be editing the music video somewhere.

How long am I going to be here? Where's Rosy? Why won't they let her in? What are they going to do to me? What the fuck is wrong with me? I'd love to go back to the real world, after a transfusion or two; but something tells me that won't be possible. I'm on a train that's ground to a halt and there hasn't been an announcement to say why. There's no way of knowing what awaits me.

Night slips beneath the slats of the badly drawn blind. I'm staying in the wheelchair because the bed scares me. I watch the tiny TV without switching it on. Someone brings me a meal in aluminium trays.

'Will I have to sleep here?'

'The doctor will let you know for sure, but I think so, Monsieur Malzieu,' replies a mask.

The cutlery is in a plastic sleeve, which the healthcare assistant rips open so I can help myself without her having to touch it. Who would have thought hell would be this clean?

Something's happening in the airlock. I recognize Rosy's silhouette: she's here at last. A breath of life. She's worried but does her best to reassure me. Her hugs are a refuge. In my last book, I invented the true story of how we met. 'The girl who disappears when you kiss her' gathers up a heart that is lying in crumbs on the ground. It belongs to the depressive inventor with a knack for feeling lovelorn. She sticks it back together, one piece at a time, with passionate patience. That's exactly what happened with us. And then today's unfathomable earthquake struck.

Rosy is perched on the bed, on the edge of the void. She's wearing her clothes from another world, the one I belonged to a few hours ago. The colours, the wind, the cars and the trees are trapped on the other side of the windowpane. I can't touch, see or hear anything any more. I make a nest with my arms and huddle inside; Rosy wraps her arms around mine.

Just then, a battalion of nurses comes into the room armed with two trays. On the first, two bottles of disinfectant solution and a chrome syringe the size of a pen. On the second, an assortment of small torture instruments and a pile of compresses. Everyone's wearing a mask. A nurse asks Rosy to leave. Another rips the patch off my sternum. 'Too high up. Pointless,' she says. My chest is wiped and rewiped with a cold product of some sort. It feels like they're preparing a target. Needles are being sterilized all over the place. I don't dare ask what they're gearing up to do; I'm frightened of the answer. A haematologist with a kind voice quietly informs me that she has to carry out 'a rather unpleasant procedure called a myelogram'. She's going to remove a bit of bone marrow from my sternum and analyse it to find out why I'm not producing blood cells.

'Put your arms by your sides, take a deep breath, try to relax and don't move.'

Now's a good time *not* to look at the harpoon they're wielding. Thick. Long. Bevelled like a dodgy pack of cards.

Two warm hands envelop mine on either side of the bed. The haematologist-with-the-kind-voice approaches. Her body over mine, weapon in hand. 'Get ready for a prick . . .'

That's putting it mildly. Get ready for an impaling, more like. She plants the thing in my sternum with both hands, using all her weight to pierce the skin and reach deep into the bone. It's like being stabbed with a banderilla. I try my hardest to breathe normally and not watch what's going on.

'And, I'm drawing it out . . .'

My torso's lifting off the bed; it's like she's trying to tear out my ribcage. Agonizing, screeching pain. I'm winded, my heart's pounding. At last the harpoon is out.

'You can breathe, it's over.'

Actually, I can't breathe right now: I'm a fucking trout who doesn't know how.

'Can you gauge the pain from zero to ten?'

'Seven, eight . . .'

I don't say ten to save face. I'm still holding hands with the nurses; I can't let go. The haematologist-with-the-kind-voice is delicately handling the carrot-shaped bone sample she has extracted from me. She slices it into strips for the biologists to analyse. Like she's preparing crudités. Then:

'Monsieur Malzieu, I'm sorry . . . We need to redo the marrow puncture.'

The nurses look at me contritely.

'Like before? The same thing?'

'Yes, there's too much blood in the sample . . . I'm worried it won't be suitable for analysis.'

There's blood all over my chest. It's still flowing under the dressing. They've sponged it, compressed it, but it won't stop. I feel like I'm witnessing my own autopsy. The haematologist prepares her second banderilla. I've been kidnapped by barbarians disguised as women with honey-sweet voices. My nerves are unravelling, my body stiffens from head to toe. The protective hands close around mine again.

'Try to think of a place you like. A beach, somewhere sunny . . .' suggests one of the nurses. What I'm thinking is that I resemble a lamb on a spit.

The haematologist looms over my chest again. Her shadow is slowly climbing up my face. I shut my eyes as tight as I can.

A second harpooning. My muscles like taut elastic bands. A second reincarnation as a trout. Breathing shallow, heart jackhammering.

'It's a brutal procedure, I'm sorry, but it's the only way we can examine bone marrow . . . Do you want a small tranquillizer, something to calm you down?'

'I wouldn't say no to a whisky and Coke.'

'Ah, sorry, we don't do that here,' the haematologist replies gently, as one might talk to a child, whereupon the battalion moves on.

The blood is taking its time to congeal under the dressing. Rosy has returned and she slips her delicate bottom on to the edge of the bed. The light from her big eyes has the effect of a strange balm.

'Try to sleep,' she whispers. I relax slightly, stroking her forearm. We kiss and it's like the inside of a meringue. I hold on to this lull in the storm, trying to think as little as possible.

A few hours later, the haematologist comes back into the room. I check straight away: she hasn't got her chrome tray.

'How are you feeling, Monsieur Malzieu?'

She chooses just the right tone of voice. Giving nothing away . . .

'The first result has come through. There are no blast cells, so you haven't got acute leukaemia.'

'Leukaemia . . .? Acute leukaemia?'

'Yes. I didn't want to mention it earlier, but that's what we feared from your blood tests.'

Acute leukaemia! When I heard those words it started raining coffins.

'We need to do further examinations to get a diagnosis and decide on your treatment. We'll know more on Tuesday.'

'But it's less serious than acute leukaemia?'

'I can't say for now. I don't have enough information. At best, it's a vitamin problem, although, saying that, with such a low blood cell count it's unlikely. At worst, you'll need to have a bone marrow transplant.'

'A bone marrow transplant? What is that?'

'Replacing your diseased bone marrow with a healthy

15

donor's. It's a tough treatment . . . But try not to worry, we're a long way off that.'

The haematologist-with-the-kind-voice is walking on egg-shells and the cracking is getting louder by the second.

'You're sure you don't want a tranquillizer to help you relax?'

'No, thank you . . .'

'Stay strong, Monsieur Malzieu. I'll see you on Tuesday.'

Declaration of war on self

12 November 2013

One by one, the analysis results deliver their verdict: 'aplastic anaemia', otherwise known as bone marrow failure. A blood disorder as serious as it is rare. Idiopathic, they call it: cause unknown. I hazard a guess that an excess of chicken nuggets and pancakes washed down with whisky and Cokes have something to do with it, but apparently not. Rock 'n' roll? Melancholy? Lovesickness? Fanatical joy? Botched sleep? Failed grief? Nutella? Nope. It's a lottery, a biological accident. It can happen to anyone and it happens to practically no one. Only a hundred cases in France. Mostly children and the elderly. I'm a collector's item.

It's remarkable to see people you hardly know distilling bad news for you in a whisper. Something ultrahuman in response to a hospital room's prison-like chill. Confined. Confounded. Confucked.

'It's not cancer, although the symptoms are identical to leukaemia. The treatment is similar, and we'll have to consider a bone marrow transplant,' the haematologist explains delicately.

I'm petrified; Rosy's eyelashes are going up and down.

'What I'm saying is, you don't have any malignant cells but your antibodies have turned against you and are attacking your healthy cells. They're treating your bone marrow as if it's a virus – we don't really know why.'

In a flash I've become my own worst enemy. The vampire sucking my blood is none other than me.

'Antibodies work like an army that is programmed to defend you. Something has made the army believe it's fighting a foreign body, whereas it's actually going after your own cells. It's what's we call an autoimmune disease.'

Bugged . . . My immune system has been hacked and now I'm self-destructing. I am my own cancer.

The peculiar redhead pallor becoming steadily more pro- nounced; those bluish stripes on the lips you get from a walk in the snow that appeared even in glaring sunshine; the feeling of having a nut where my lungs should be; always being the only one who was cold – so *that's* what it was . . . But there's no time to absorb the shock. I have to tell my family. The thought of phoning my dad and my sister terrifies me. I don't know how to explain this surreal, real diagnosis.

They've taken phials and phials of blood, stuck harpoons in my back for another bone marrow biopsy and at last I'm allowed to go home. Provided I come back at least once a week for a transfusion. From now on, I'll need other people's blood to stay alive. It's official: I've turned into a vampire.

To return to the land of the living, I need a bone marrow transplant. The treatment's tough, too tough in some cases. On the internet they say you can die.

Extra-terrestrial attack

14 November 2013

I ask loads of questions, of myself and other people. I don't always understand the answers. Bone marrow isn't an organ, so you can't picture it. A heart or kidney transplant is frightening, but you know what it is. In my case, it's a hazy fear. A nebulous danger like an extra-terrestrial attack.

People tend to confuse bone marrow with the spinal cord. Before the diagnosis I couldn't have told you that bone marrow produces blood cells. Turns out it's every bit as vital as the heart.

My body is now a minefield. To avoid going boom while I'm waiting for a transplant, I must obey three laws, just like Jack in *The Cuckoo-Clock Heart*:

1. No strenuous physical activities (because of the lack of oxygen in my blood)
2. Avoid public places, kissing and physical contact of any kind with pretty much everyone (because of my weakened immune system)

3. And above all, never, ever, bang into anything (to reduce the risk of a haemorrhage)

Hell, in other words, for someone who likes rolling around on the ground and crowd surfing. Goodbye concerts (mine and other people's), mates, whisky bars, the cinema, cycling, bombing it on a skateboard, trips down south with the family, travelling, making life up as I go along, freedom . . . Even cleaning my teeth with a brush is too dangerous. From now on, it's antibacterial gel, mouthwash and time spent alone. As for the idea of becoming a dad . . . I'll have to save myself first.

The vampire of Rue de Bretagne

15 November 2013

It's strange walking around my *quartier* the way I used to when everything was all right. Talking about football and poetry with the newsagent as if nothing is amiss. It's trickier with the pharmacists who turn pale as they read my prescriptions: '. . . administered for the treatment of a recognized long-term illness.

'No one knows I'm a vampire. I haven't turned into a bat yet. I still appear in mirrors. I look like a ghost in a woolly hat, but my reflection's still there. The sight of a crucifix doesn't make me run for the hills, maybe because I'm already out of breath as it is. I'm not doing weird stuff at double speed like in the movies. But I am a real vampire: I need other people's blood to stay alive. And I'm snowflake-white to look at too.

Since I'm a prisoner of my own body, I must learn to escape into my thoughts more than ever before. Organize my resistance by mobilizing the resources of my imagination. I'm going to work hard at my dream of getting out of this. I'll need forged-iron will. The stuff of marathon runners. Stride after stride. Rhythm and perseverance. Strike a balance between monk-like rigour and creative fantasy. Learn to mess about creatively within the austere limits of the curfew I must now respect. Measure out hope one day at a time. Transform total darkness into a star-spangled night. Pluck the moon from the sky in the morning and have it back in place by dusk.

A job for a neo-vampire.

Science-fiction gardening

Transplanting bone marrow is a bit like science-fiction garden-ing. First, find a compatible donor, in other words a person whose genetic code – or HLA* – is identical to yours. There's a one in four chance that my sister possesses the famous seeds that could make my cells grow back again. Otherwise it's the biological lottery of the worldwide donor register. But then the odds increase to one in a million.

Say we find it. Before carrying out the transplant, they would have to uproot my diseased bone marrow. Make room to accom-modate the new graft. Hence chemotherapy and radiotherapy. Only then will my body be ready to receive the famous stem cells that are said to be 'haematopoietic'. These magic beans will pass through my veins and lodge themselves deep in my bones. And if all goes well (no rejection or complications), a few months later I'll become a chimeric being: half me, half

---

* HLA – the human leukocyte antigen – is the unique immunological ID card we all possess.

someone else. A rebirth, but with the help of a new biological parent. I could even change blood groups.

The transplant process will be slow. For the seed cells to grow, I'll have to stay in a greenhouse – a sterile room. And wait patiently for the cells' springtime, in the haemato-poetic hope of budding again.

They won't be giving me a clockwork heart in place of a frozen one, but, just like *The Boy with the Cuckoo-Clock Heart*, it's a matter of life or death. This time reality surpasses (science) fiction.

Dame Oclès

25 November 2013

My big little sister is going to do a blood test for me. She wants to give me some of her bone marrow and the surge of affection breaks my heart. I don't want to imagine her being surgically pincered by crabs in white coats. I know they'll be gentle but I can't bear the idea of her getting hurt.

Dad phoned, his sadness as heavy as an anvil. His speech has slowed, like a record played at the wrong speed. But his voice is still warm and comforting. A real dad-voice. Night falls and the vampire in pyjamas comes into his own. Rosy has fallen asleep with her make-up on and only one sock. Watching her fidget in her sleep helps me block out reality for a few moments.

Then I settle down in my favourite chair. My refuge, my cabin, my chapel of creation. From here, I have an uninterrupted view over the invisible kingdom, the only place I can live without restrictions. Here, I can invent stories and teach the children I'd like to have how to skateboard. Or eat cakes without making a sound, or pick up the wrong bottle in the dark and give myself a port mouthwash. I burrow into my night nest. And end up taking a sleeping pill so I'll fall asleep before dawn – it's very bad for a vampire's health to be awake in broad daylight. I slip my frozen feet beside Rosy's hot-water bottle body and drop off at last.

In the middle of a dream, my nose starts bleeding. I'm woken by the taste of blood in my mouth. The white pillow is stained red. Through the window the stars are losing their colour. Nearly day. It's a monumental struggle to get out of bed; my body is glued to the mattress. I haul myself up like a weightlifter and go in search of something to patch myself up. The compresses get redder and redder; it won't stop. I'm knocked out by the anaemia and the pills. I just want to get back to my dream. I'm dizzy and freezing cold.

A noise makes me jump. I lift my head and catch my reflection in the bedroom mirror. I still can't stem the flow of blood. No compresses left. No more Coalgan either, to stop the bleeding.

Another rasping sound behind me. This time I turn around. A shadow moves. Rosy? I glance at the bed: she's huddled under the duvet. Another noise – in the bathroom this time. Metallic, as if someone's just broken something. I open the door, carefully so it doesn't squeak, and slip into the room. The noise is louder. That felt like a breath on my shoulder. Biting cold. I turn on the tap to splash some water over my face.

'Well I never – a vampire in pyjamas!' says a silky voice.

I turn. A female figure is draped in my bath. She's filing her nails with a sword. A mane of glowing red hair cascades over translucent shoulders. Her eyelashes are long and fake-looking. A slash of eyeliner holds my gaze.

'I didn't think you'd be so small . . .'

Her voice sounds like the woman who does the pre-recorded announcements on station platforms.

'I'll have to aim well to cut off your head.'

She glides the face of the blade against my cheek.

'Who are you and—'

She cuts me off: 'I am Dame Oclès.'

'Dame who?'

'Oclès . . . Dame Oclès. You know! I've got a famous sword,' she says, proudly tapping the metal blade.

'Dame Oclès . . . Doesn't ring a bell.'

'What do you mean, "Doesn't ring a bell"?'

'Nope, it doesn't ring a bell.'

'Well, you'll get to know me soon enough, because from now on, I go where you go,' she says, lifting her sword above my head.

Her lips are redder than haemoglobin, as if she's drunk blood as meticulously as other women put on make-up. She's smoking a slim cigarette of the Vogue variety and using my sink as an ashtray. Like the prow of an elegant galleon, her bosom proudly bears the black standard of her décolleté. That could have your eye out – but in a good way.

'Um, right, if you want to stay in the bathroom that's fine, but I'm going back to bed.'

'Sooner or later you'll have to confront me. There's no escaping our little face-off,' she says, guiding the freezing blade over the nape of my neck.

Is fear giving me hallucinations? Or is it the lack of oxygen in my blood? Disturbed by this vision, I go back to bed with the taste of metal in my mouth.

★

Next morning, I recall my dream with the clarity of a memory. My pillow really is stained with blood. But Dame Oclès isn't in the bath any more and I can almost shower in peace. Mind you, the showerhead gets heavier and heavier; the simple effort of holding it over my head wears me out. I'm obsessed with last night. I feel the presence of Dame Oclès in the lift, in the back seat of the taxi . . . Everywhere.

But I try to keep forging ahead. Today, I'm meeting people at a cinema to see a screening of the film. I've waited six years for this moment. We've fought tooth and nail to get it on, so showing off *Jack and the Cuckoo-Clock Heart* is a proud moment. And yet . . . It's a bizarre sensation, watching a film that was shot inside your own heart.

My film colleagues are walking on invisible eggshells because of my vampire problem. It's touching and embarrassing at the same time. I hold my producer in my arms for six seconds. Six years of work, of magical twists and turns and dramas combine in that hug – without us saying a word. A precious précis. Then a taxi pootles into view in the rain, and I leave the same way I came.

I know I'm going to be robbed of much of the joy associated with the release of this film. I have to learn to make do with leftovers from the treasure trove. I am beginning to face facts, but now a race within a race has begun to unfold: will I be able to promote this film properly? It's possible I'll be admitted to the sterile room before its release . . .

A countdown has started. Somehow or other, I have to make it to 5 February. This film is my beating pulse. My blood flows in every shot. As a point of honour, whatever happens, I won't let myself slide into bitterness. But to watch the dream I've been tirelessly working towards vanishing into thin air would be a terrible blow.

My heart says yes, my head says yes, the rest of my body shrugs. The fact is, as things stand, we don't have a donor.

The vampire of love

Illness magnetizes love and turns the heart into a sieve, simultaneously. My heart was pierced at birth. But since the diagnosis it's even worse. This particular vampire needs love as well as blood. Rosy is my consenting prey. 'I wish you didn't have to suffer,' I say, as I devour her. I don't tell her about Dame Oclès, so as not to worry her, but I know she's haunted by her too in her own way.

Meanwhile, the carnage is confirmed. The severe lack of red blood cells, the 'anaemia', has turned off the oxygen tap to my whole body. My muscles are tired before they're even used. Getting dressed makes me feel like an old-age sumo wrestler. The platelets are still melting away too; my blood barely clots any more. My nose erupts volcanically completely out of the blue. As if the Invisible Man clocks me one from time to time. As for my white blood cells, they're turning transparent. That means I'm ideal prey for viruses; I've got no immune system to fight them off.

I'm going to need blood. More and more blood, more and more frequently. As biting isn't really my style, I go to hospital a lot.

Self-made superhero

A journalist and his film crew come to interview me at home about the film. When one of them sneezes I hold my breath. It doesn't protect me in any way, but it's instinctive.

In minutes, they've turned my apartment into a mini-television studio. I'm sitting on the sofa, just as I do when the nurse comes to take my blood. They've hooked me up to a lapel mic and the word-sample trickles out of me convivially. It's fun to play at being my other self. The man I was last month. They're making my job easy because in their eyes I'm a director, not a patient.

The interview is over, the crew pack up their toys. I'm emptied, just like after a medical examination, but it's done me good to talk about a cuckoo-clock transplant instead of bone marrow, blood cells and hospital.

Then Joann Sfar drops by with pancakes and a jar of Nutella. He asks very precise questions and listens equally carefully to my answers. It's relaxing not to have to explain everything over and over again. Kind gestures warm my heart but what helps me most at the moment is people who really listen.

His conclusion, washed down with two *crêpes au Nutella* and a Coke, is as follows: 'You've got no choice: you have to become a self-made superhero. It'll make a good story one day, even if you have a rough old time along the way.'

That's something to hold on to.

Disguised as myself

'I've never been this sad and happy at the same time,' says my character in the film. That pretty well sums up my life these days. Sunday spent watching my own movie on the big screen in the *Forum des images* packed with mates, and Monday trapped in hospital. Day and night. Contrasts and metamorphoses.

Today I pretended I wasn't ill and I loved it. The slightest kiss is more dangerous for me than a yomp in the equatorial jungle, but I love living dangerously. A tableful of friends eating chips as night falls. Warming words and fruit-juice cocktails. I would have loved a drop of whisky. What a strange melancholic luxury to celebrate the film's release with people who don't know about my 'health problem'. I'm a ghost disguised as myself. And for now you can't see the join.

But midnight sounds and the vampire-me must get back into his pyjamas. Tomorrow it's a bone marrow biopsy and blood transfusions. Oh, and whatever you do, make sure you don't go to pieces. I try to stock up on joy during my night out. I'll need it if I'm to scale tomorrow morning's medical glacier.

A bloody marrow-thon

9 December 2013

You can recognize the route to the hospital by the cheery business outlets scattered round about. The entrance is just after the third funeral parlour on the right. The hospital building looks like a large sad school full of pupils who've been kept behind for bad behaviour. There's a chapel so people can cry in peace and a newsagent's where you can buy sweets and a copy of *L'Équipe*. Read the football scores, have a quick pray and munch on a Mars bar.

I'm going to have my platelets changed. I go with the flow these days. Got no choice. Virtually all the clotting particles in my blood have liquefied. If I stroke a hedgehog with the tips of my fingers I'll get a bruise right up to my elbow.

But it seems the centre of gravity has shifted today. The bone marrow biopsy reveals a slight improvement. A few crumbs of comfort, perhaps. It may be possible to get my system back on track with a less arduous treatment than a transplant. The principle: wipe out the antibodies that are attacking my bone marrow with anti-lymphocyte globulin (ALG), an equivalent to chemotherapy derived from horse or rabbit proteins. Once my antibodies are out of harm's way, my bone marrow cells may grow back. Then, we'll have to keep my antibodies undercooked for a few months; an immunosuppressant drug called ciclosporin will see to that. The hope is that during their enforced sleep, my antibodies will forget to confuse my cells with a virus and I'll stop self-destructing. Reboot. Turn it off, and hope it turns back on again. Just like when your computer has frozen, you gamble on 'restart' solving the problem.

The downside of the treatment is that my whole immune system will be weakened once again. I'll be even more vulnerable to infection, hence the sterile room. The film's coming out in less than two months. They want me to agree to various interviews but I don't know how long I can delay going into hospital. I've got publicists on the phone, doctors, then publicists again . . . I have to hold out.

There's a fifty-fifty chance that the immunosuppressant treatment will be enough to cure me. So a chance, a big 'maybe' wedged in the vice as it turns. Because if the transplant route becomes the only option, we still don't have a donor. The search has been widened to the worldwide register but, for now, they can't find a matching genetic code for a Lorrain-Spanish-Oranian hybrid from Montpellier. My sister isn't compatible either. She sounded sad on the phone. She told me three times that she was sure she would be. She wanted it so much she had convinced herself she was.

All the while, red cells are deserting my blood the way football fans desert a stadium after a defeat. Bowed heads and self-deluded bleats about the referee are the order of the day. My blood count is dropping like the temperature; these are the shortest days of the year . . . but perhaps the longest of my life. As for the transfusion rate, that's on the rise.

Today, I'm as tired as my results are low. My arm is covered in little red marks. They are petechiae, sort of mini-haemorrhages caused by the lack of platelets. 'Give up.' Just saying the words leaves a nasty taste in my mouth.

I'm frightened of going into the bathroom and finding Dame Oclès there. I thank the night for growing a fairy form in my bed with arms as soft as warm croissants. If you live with Rosy, it's like adopting a magical animal. I feel like all seven dwarves rolled into one, watching Snow White turn dust into sparkles. Day and night she fights at my side. Listens. Gives me a boost. Encourages. Never drops her guard. Protects my imaginary kingdom, protects the flame that keeps me alive.

Night's colours are fading. I'm going to try and dream about clockwork bone marrow transplanted by a magician. Just wind it up every morning and it makes new cells. I'd give the key to Rosy.

Gravity

15 December 2013

The emotional pile-up continues. This is a rollercoaster ride in a knackered old carriage with no safety bar: I've found out I have to spend the Christmas holidays in hospital. My white blood cells are melting like ice cubes in a bonfire; the risk of infection is growing by the day. The doctors want to protect me by bringing my admission to the sterile room forward. Inside, I'll be given the famous anti-lymphocyte horse remedy and the ciclosporin. If all goes well, I'll be out three weeks later. It's looking increasingly likely I won't be able to promote the film; it comes out on 5 February and the bulk of the promo work starts around 15 January. I have to explain as much to all the experts I talk to, some of whom fail to understand the gravity of the situation or what this film means to me. I decide to take control of my fate just for a moment: I want to spend Christmas with my family. I'll go into the sterile room after that.

Professionally, I'm starting to frighten people. So it's almost comforting to return to the hospital and pour myself into the nurses' hypodermic arms. Nestle in their empathy. Their eyes don't give anything away, so I can, through them, picture myself as healthy. Mobiles and melodious music are wafted over my head to try and make me unwind, as if I were a baby. And it works a bit. Best to let myself slide into this fuzzy embrace. Wait for tomorrow and the quiet weekend to follow. All being well, I've nothing medical to do until Monday. An eternity for a vampire in pyjamas.

I'm discovering that being ill sorts the people you think of as friends into different categories. Having a severe health problem is remarkably similar to being successful: it changes people's behaviour towards you. A dip in illness's darkroom reveals their true colours. The considerate, the clumsy, the brave, the solid . . . The sordid too. Those who jump ship at the height of the storm, even though it's provided them with food and shelter for years. Those who stop working with you and ask you to call 'when you're better'. Those who are waiting to see whether you get out of this, or not, before coming aboard again. Those who abandon, those who betray. They don't all know they're doing it perhaps, but they're pushing me into the arms of Dame Oclès.

There are also people who do whatever it takes to encourage you, who 'believe'. Those who listen, those who offer what they can, those who don't see me as a vampire. And those who know perfectly well I am one but would never stoop to discrimination. Those who get the creative juices flowing. Or any sort of juices.

I've officially been a vampire for a month, but probably ill for much longer. I did bleed a lot when I threw myself into the crowd during last year's concerts. After walking up a flight of stairs my calves would hurt as if I'd just climbed the Col du Tourmalet.* I always had an impressive collection of bruises too.

Today, I'm going for a skate like an elderly child. Very gently, with gloves on and a woolly hat pulled down over my ears. I'm like a dog on a leash: mustn't go too far, mustn't pull too hard. One bit of gravel jammed in a wheel and I'll turn into a haemoglobin garden sprinkler. I think about it enough to stop myself going any faster. But not too much, so I don't just freeze up.

I'm a bear waking up from hibernation, my senses are numb and hyper-receptive at the same time. I'm frightened of the cold and of people, but I hear the colours of the setting sun throbbing in the mist. I want to take a photo of it all, and bag up the fresh air as a souvenir.

---

* The Pyrenean mountain pass renowned for its sheer slopes, which make for a mythic ascent in the Tour de France.

Manon or Pierre

To keep my insomnia company I've adopted a hedgehog. I wanted a real one but he's plastic because of the fleas. I put him on my shoulder and we stroll around my 35 square metres. We look at cars out of the window. This animal knows the art of self-preservation, so he protects me too. I've been doing better since I got him. He's not even that snazzy, as hedgehogs go, but still . . .

In the midnight hours, when I manage to unwind, I picture a spring day and me skating in a pullover with my brand-new bone marrow. Just breezy! Ah, never underestimate the importance of the frivolous daydream.

Rosy is not in denial about the illness, which makes her hope all the more restorative. Her body is uncannily like a mammilla tree, which only produces two fruit in a lifetime. It's said that if you fall asleep in its branches, you'll wake up in love. True story . . . When I'm in hospital and it's time for her to head off into the night, I think I'll unscrew her bosoms. I'll put them on my bedside table and when I feel particularly anxious I can squeeze them like two oranges. I'll hide them in the little cup-board next to the bed and in the morning she can come and pick them up on her way to work.

We're managing to laugh in Dame Oclès' face. We've been playing ping-pong on the sitting-room table. Our togetherness always bubbles up to the surface. We're resistance fighters armed with affection. We're helping each other, like a mini-family. Per-haps because Christmas is coming or because I'm ill or because it feels good to be stuck to one another all this time, we've talked about babies. The great post-war 'maybe'. If I win the war, that is . . .

Rosy's frightened of giving birth. She's not good with pain. Brave, but really not good with pain. She cries swallowing an aspirin. So we've decided to have a very premature baby. It'll be born at six weeks, like a tiny rabbit. No bigger than a kiwi fruit. I'll invent a sort of aquarium-incubator and we'll put it on the shelf between the popcorn maker and the record player. Manon or Pierre will grow before our very eyes, transparently. Friends who come round will say, 'Oh, what a nice turtle . . . Have you got a 3D printer? What is it? Some kind of exotic fruit?' And we'll proudly reply, 'It's Manon or Pierre. If you want to smoke, kindly leave the room.'

Have yourself a merry scary Christmas

23 December 2013

I've got less than 7 grams of haemoglobin in my blood. This morning, getting out of the shower, I was so weak I thought I was going to rub myself out with the towel.

But Rosy and I are still giving ourselves a proper romantic Christmas. Which is basically like doing a last slow dance on the moon, when the oxygen tanks are empty, the spaceship's broken and no one knows how to get home. Except it's actually given me an oxygen *boost*.

We've only just finished the mad dash to buy Christmas presents. I filled a sports bag as big as Father Christmas's sack, and a burly Father Christmas at that. Later this afternoon I'm catching a train to spend Christmas with my family. I've got to wear a mask on the journey, but it's a small price to pay for returning to my childhood home. Before that, I must go to the hospital for a blood test.

I arrive at the reception desk, where they've decked the halls with scraps of tinsel. A woman with a hole in the head and a sphincter for a heart begins the merry scary Christmas hostilities.

Yes, I've got all the appointment details in an email on my phone and yes, it's the festive season, but she needs '*le papier*'. I show her my name and the name of the doctor who works on the floor above, but she wants '*le papier*'. Not to file away or anything; no, just because she must always see '*le papier*'.

Eventually, the haematologist-with-the-kind-voice sees me. She tells me I won't be going into the glass bubble on Thursday as planned. That, in fact, I might not be going in at all. It seems I have an ungenerous gene. And it could be responsible for this whole sorry fuck-up. It's a rare genetic condition. A disorder that can't be treated with anti-lymphocyte globulin and ciclosporin. This thingamajig anaemia could attack other parts of my body, cause cancer and, most significantly, affect other members of my family. As for my dream of having kids, it's quietly fading away. They need to double-check this finding with a bone marrow biopsy by harpoon, in the thigh this time. If the diagnosis is confirmed, we're back to square one: a bone marrow transplant, donor willing. Fancy depending on an organ you can't get hold of.

I go home on foot. I need the walk. The dry cold biting the tips of my ears reminds me I'm alive. I'm wiped out by the time I reach the third floor of my apartment block. I sit down and eat the chocolate decorations from the mini-Christmas tree. All of them. I put an Elvis record on the turntable. Dame Oclès is lounging on my bed. I am at her mercy. I feel sorry for myself.

But it's still Christmas. My gums bled after we opened presents this evening. As if I'd bitten into the jugular of some poor innocent victim. I was frightened. I didn't let on. Dad came to get some things out of the room where I'm supposed to be sleeping – rather than writing – and he found me holding a compress oozing blood. He was as loving as two parents rolled into one. I cried like two children rolled into one. Then the bleeding stopped. I'm wondering if I'm going to wake up dead tomorrow morning. Or find I've grown fangs. Or both.

Before my gums started to bleed, I was granted a proper family Christmas Eve. Laughter, surprises and cake. The simple joy of giving and receiving presents. The extraordinary ordinary. I took love in and I gave love out, trying to push this marrow-thon business to one side. I think we pulled it off.

The return of Dame Oclès

27 December 2013

Hugs on the platform, a bag stuffed with presents, eyelids like a portcullis. Keeping the tears locked away inside my skull. And wearing a surgical mask of course. Must have swallowed some butterflies. I'm scared I won't see them again. The whole family, my lovely nieces, the band. I'm wearing a big kid's hat and a warm jacket, though it's not that cold. All I'm missing is a pair of bloody skis. Actually, I wouldn't mind seeing the mountains again. Taking off those plastic robot shoes, then eating a pancake. Bare feet on a carpet soggy with melted snow. Wrapping up warm and sitting by a fireside drying socks. Talking bumps and bruises. And wind chill factors.

The train will cut through the valley. I know its scissoring course by heart. Even the order the clouds have gathered themselves in seems familiar. Dame Oclès is sitting on the third step of the TGV's automatic door. A pair of black trousers moulded to her arse as if she's just dipped her legs in a pool of oil. Her high heels are so pointy she could impale the whole carriage on them. I shiver feverishly when she bats her wing-lids.

'Hey, do you know which way the buffet car is?'

'I think it's closed . . .'

'I'm bloody starving. Aren't you hungry?'

'No, I'm fine, thanks.'

'Eh? Can't understand a word you're saying in that stupid bloody mask. Take it off.'

I pretend I'm not listening and check my mask is protecting my face by carefully pinching it over my nose.

'Listen, you're done for anyway. Don't you want to go out with a bang? They're ruining the release of your film, they're fucking up your body with their drugs and it's making your family cry. Are you just going to wait around like this until the end?'

'I'll get over this, even if it takes time.'

'Ah! But you know you won't, deep down . . . Be honest with me.'

'I am.'

'Oh yeah . . . If not with me, try and be honest with yourself at least.'

'I'm—'

She cuts me off. 'Look, come with me. Don't you want to see the finest breasts in the galaxy before you're put in a sterile room?'

'I've already seen them.'

'Ah, you've no idea, pal . . . If you won't think of yourself, at least think of the people who are going to watch you dwindle to nothing. You'll make them suffer. Or you could skip all that and choose to go with joyful dignity and a bit of panache!'

She points her gleaming sword at my nose.

'Or maybe you prefer the hospital's vegetable soup and being woken up by those poor girls jabbing you with their needles . . . And in their shapeless blouses too, oh dear! Anyway, it's your call. You coming to the buffet car with me?'

'I've already eaten.'

Dame Oclès shrugs her sublime shoulders, folds her willowy body up the steps and disappears.

Happy Blue Year!

31 December 2013

The net I'm caught in is tightening: it's chainmail now. Heavy-metal hell. I'm grappling with doubts of steel. My suit of armour is rebelling and destroying me from the inside.

I do want to fight. These are not the ramblings of death; hyper-life is what keeps me going, and always has done. I want to fight. But not if it's a lost cause. Not if it's rigged at a chromosomal level and even a successful transplant of mammoth proportions would only be a reprieve. I'm not sure I want to board that particular train. I'm waiting for a piece of good news, an injection of something celestial, a *je ne sais quoi* of light at the end of the tunnel. In this icy impenetrable fog, my heart is breaking. Every phone call to my dad or my sister turns my head into a goldfish bowl of tears that spills over the minute I hang up. I love life too much to accept the idea of death. I'm blown away that this illness might blow me away.

Rosy remains almost unflappable. She's a warrior armed with weapons of kindness. Her heart is as big as a station clock. I see her fighting to slow down time when the fast-forward feeling is making me anxious, and speed time up when it's dragging.

I played her a new tune today: 'The Song of the Bad Swan'. For the first time, I've touched on my present situation: a little musical offering in a children's folk-gospel style. No one else has heard it. Rosy has watched me bleed, receive transfusions, be impaled with needles from head to toe and she's never let it throw her. But when I started to sing, she burst into tears. The incredible dam she has built up day by day to protect us gave way. Condensed fear burst forth down her cheeks. Melancholic panic. I had a hell of a job calming her down. Hugs and sweet nothings did the trick in the end. I was sorry for causing her eyes to break their banks like that, but pleased I could console her for once, instead of the other way round. That she could count on me. Afterwards, we laughed, I played silly songs on the guitar and we got dressed up for our mini-New Year's Eve at home. I don't know what she put in those pancakes, but I spent the evening as happy as a man who doesn't know his bone marrow from his garden marrow.

On this 31 December at midnight, we both phoned our families to wish them happy new year. Happy blue year in my case. It was also my dad's seventy-fifth birthday. I feel I'm getting older than him by the day. I'm looking after his mental health because his little boy is ill. Neither of us has a mummy any more; he hasn't had one for ages. Losing a child must be even worse. I try to reassure him, even when I'm not reassured myself. He's scared. So scared that sometimes he borders on denial. It's his way of dealing with hope. What's left unsaid hurts us both, but the epic vitality of our father–son connection holds firm.

The man who looked distinguished in tracksuit bottoms

3 January 2014

It's back to the hellish routine: schlepping to and from the outpatient clinic. Dame Oclès follows me like my shadow now. Everywhere, all the time. She watches me in the shower, chuckles when I take too long to get dressed. Her favourite moment when we go to the haematology department is walking past the death parlours on Rue Saint-Jacques. She shrieks with delight at the sight of the engraved marble slabs. Like a teenage girl in a department store. 'Which one's your favourite? Oh my god, that would *so* suit you!' she says, pointing to a vintage-looking coffin that looks second-hand. 'It's very vampire. You should probably reserve it, don't you think?'

We amble like two half-dead lovers along the little road reserved for ambulances that runs adjacent to the Achard building, the huge sad school where I go for lessons in survival. I call the lift; it looks like a mini-hospital room that moves. We reach the fifth floor. Shiver-inducing words everywhere: Haematology, Oncology, Immunology. Mybodyowesmeanapology. Lame jokes help clear my mind for a moment.

The waiting room. Magazines showing off the most realistic wigs on the market. Old people who are, in fact, younger than me. We recognize each other by the plasters on our arms. The transfusion gang. We end up greeting each other like friendly neighbours, thanks to our frequent encounters here.

It's rare to meet people who look distinguished in tracksuit bottoms. It happened to me this afternoon. In my transfusion room. A vampire of about seventy wearing smart city shoes from another life. And curious fleeced sportswear designed to give his tired body some comfort. There was delicate determination and dignity in the way he asked the nurses to help him take off the shoes.

Then the haematologist arrived. Subdued, voice volume turned right down. They talked about how much time he has left, what he's still able to do. The different ways he might die. I didn't dare watch any more. I listened without listening. Colossal difficulties revealed themselves with every syllable she uttered. I left the room to let them utter secrets without secrecy, words as hard as flint. When they had finished, I went back in. He still looked distinguished in his tracksuit bottoms; his shoes were placed at the foot of the bed. He was dozing and his sleep invaded the room like a soothing balm. I fell asleep myself. I hope he was able to dream.

When he stood up, as carefully as one might unfold porcelain sheets, he thanked me for my tact with a voice like a songless Leonard Cohen. The ambulance men took him away. Compassionate policemen leading away a caring crook. They closed the door behind them and I felt like the weakest man in the world.

★

Dame Oclès whispers in my ear that my haemoglobin levels are lower than the man who looked distinguished in tracksuit bottoms. It's true.

I try reading Walt Whitman to give me the courage not to listen to her. I can still see her by the window, slicing shadows with her sword. I take a newspaper out of my bag and pretend it's a magic shield. The paper is bigger than the Whitman, and easier to read. My best weapons for repelling Dame Oclès remain humour and poetry. The minute I laugh or delight in something, I give her the slip. When the anaemia pummels my brain so much that I can't read or write, there's always anger. And when I'm too tired to get angry, I play the ukulele.

Two nurses enter the room smiling. The sight of a china-white vampire reading *L'Équipe* and wearing a pair of oversized sunglasses mid-transfusion makes them laugh. Every time I see new blood passing through the plastic tube on its way to my veins, I feel like God's feeding me. A human God, who dropped by on his way home from work with a little gift for me. Today, once again, I'm being kept alive by an anonymous person and by the medical staff who convey the blood from his or her veins to mine.

In the room next door I overhear:

'You know you've got a myelogram today?'

'I know, I know . . . Someone's going to suck out my soul again.'

The man's voice seems to be emanating from the Whitman book. Describing the 'rather unpleasant procedure' so perfectly. We're all in the same boat here. Even poet-ghosts must suffer harpoon fishing in the sternum.

I'm as tense as a bowstring. After him, it's my turn. 'O Captain! My Captain!' May your poetic power ease the pain . . .

'Monsieur Malzieu? You're next . . .' Astonishingly, sharing the experience of a myelogram with Walt Whitman doesn't make me any braver. Having to endure this procedure all over again petrifies me. Two junior doctors come towards me with a thick needle called a trocar. I'm tempted to do a Wolverine from the first *X-Men* film: leap out of bed at double speed, dodge the needle and pin the doctor to the wall. But I'm not Wolverine.

The procedure is short and sharp. Two spells of ten-second torture and then stillness. Dressing applied, heartbeat slowing. Lots of pain, how much gain? Now I must wait for the verdict once again.

The nurses and the doctors are sweet; their habit of popping their heads round the door to make sure that 'everything's all right' cushions the panic. I haven't known such comfort in solitude since I had chickenpox. When my mum would turn up in my room with broth with pasta shapes.

In the haematology department of Hôpital Cochin, even the most beautiful nurses wear plastic granny shoes and everyone's disguised as a crumpled ghost. The music from the infusion pumps is a symphony of clock-radio alarm tones from the eighties. The yellow sheets embroidered 'Hôpitaux de Paris' are the same colour as urine, probably so you can piss in them undercover. But you get a five-star château welcome.

I'm starting to feel close to them all. What impresses me is their patience and their ability to listen. They walk tall among the lumbering shadows that wander the hospital corridors. They steer lifeboats with tiny rudders through storms of distress. They're beautiful people.

I still believe in the Marrow Fairy but doubts are setting in. Will they find a donor or have they already combed the whole worldwide register? The answers from my haematologist are vague. She juggles hope as carefully as you would fine-china juggling balls. Mustn't drop it . . .

I left the outpatient clinic on the arm of my beloved. An OAP in tight jeans. An invisible wind was blowing hard in the hospital corridor, I held on to her with all my miniature might. The medication they gave me to prevent allergic reactions has rendered me dead on my feet. I'm so tired.

If I do get out of this, I'll become a different man. I can already feel the metamorphosis at work. I've spent a lifetime dreaming of chimeras, giants, amorous monsters and sirens, and here I am fighting for a return to 'normality'. The most intense fairy tale there is. To linger in a bookshop and think of nothing more than finding a good book. Not worrying about that bloke who's coughing or when I'm due to take my pills, just quietly losing myself. I've always loved to dream big; right now I just want to live like everyone else.

Star Wars

15 January 2014

Today's the day I get the verdict about the genetic condition. What terrifies me is the thought that other members of my family might be affected.

I arrive at another vast illness supermarket known as Hôpital Saint-Louis. As you go in, there's a charming boutique selling wigs and prosthetic breasts. Further along, a station concourse with a board showing different medical departments instead of towns and departure times. No trains, just people whiter than sheets going off the rails, as far as their mobile drips will take them. They look like zombies doing their weekly Casino shop.

Of course I have to register my arrival. An arsenal of forms, files and receptionists. It's like a deathly Jobcentre. Now, I admit I'm rubbish at paperwork. This time I've forgotten to bring my ID card. When you're boarding a flight to Réunion Island, I understand why they check it. When you're coming to see a doctor about a serious illness I struggle, to be honest. I've got my bank card and the name on it matches the details of the appointment, but no, they need my ID card. Just in case a joker thinks, 'Brilliant! I'm going to hang about in a hospital reception for an hour and a half and pretend to be him, ha, ha . . .'

I'm visiting a prison, maybe a cemetery. Unless it's a fucking magic trampoline. In the waiting room, my heart leaps into my throat when I read the information pamphlet about the genetic condition in question. If I've got it, my far from rosy prognosis will have upped sticks and moved to a brand-new location even further from rosy. I wait my turn to see the professor from the bone marrow transplant unit. If I make it that far, he'll be in charge of the operations.

I'm received by an extraordinary human being hidden behind a white coat who speaks to me quite normally. He's an aplasia* specialist who is an expert in empathy. Or the other way round. Present, alert, concerned, clear, encouraging and you understand what he's saying. No jargon. No lecturing. Just the science. He's a specialist in Humane Sciences. Of course, had he given me bad news I might not have been such a fan. There is no genetic problem, according to the biopsy. My illness won't affect other members of my family. So, I'm not a congenital vampire. Nor am I highly disposed to multiple and varied cancers. The sword of Dame Oclès, whose blade I could feel getting rusty on my neck, recedes slightly. There are two potential anti-lymphocytic treatments available to us before the transplant stage. I've just put some time between me and the completion of the Death

---

* Aplasia is the state in which the impatient inpatient finds himself without white blood cells and thus confined to a sterile room to avoid the risk of infection.

Star. Months, years perhaps, or – you never know – a whole lifetime.

I've offered to make a deal with the professor. I'll lock myself away in a sterile room, I'll take all the necessary immuno-suppressant drugs, I'll eat war rations, I'll wear the paper uniform they give to the bedridden, but I'll do so *after* the film's release on 5 February.

They say that when you cut off a samurai's head, he carries on fighting for a few seconds. It also applies to zombies and chickens. Whatever happens next, I'll continue to exist for the duration of a ninety-minute film in 3D.

Telephoning my father and sister to tell them they're safe fills me with a deep muted joy, like a tree that can feel the sap circulating in its roots. A new impulse to fight is growing inside me. I will go head-to-head with Dame Oclès.

The hospital and its ghosts

22 January 2014

Transplant. No transplant. Hospitalised. Not hospitalised. Transplant. Yes. No. Maybe. Definitely. Now. Later. Immediately! It's nerve-shredding, this.

My haematologist runs through the latest test results.

'We won't be able to wait until 5 February to bring you in: your white blood cell count is too low. You run the risk of getting an infection, which would push back the treatment date still further . . . I know it's difficult for you with your film coming out, but it's getting much too risky now.'

There's a lullaby lilt to her words that's designed to put children to sleep. It doesn't work so well on vampires.

'There's only two weeks to go, but they're the most important. The preview, press, screenings in various cinemas on the day of the release. And I feel good, a bit tired, yeah, but I'll be able to relax all I want afterwards . . . The professor from Saint-Louis says it's OK.'

'Yes, but he doesn't follow your case on a day-to-day basis, and since you saw him your bloods have dropped. The risk of infection is increasing. It's dangerous to be out of hospital for that long.'

'It's very important to me that I see this film through to the end. I'll come in on the morning of the sixth if need be . . .'

'I understand. I'll talk to the rest of the team and let you know.'

The haematologist-with-the-kind-voice says goodbye faster than her shadow. I can see she's trying to accommodate me and being as sensitive as she possibly can, but that she also has difficult decisions to make. She's like a teacher duty-bound to punish a pupil she's fond of. I know she drowned me in bad news, but I still like her. I've got a bit attached actually, like an idiot.

The phone rings. It's my producer. I have to confirm the date for *Le Grand Journal** and various other interviews. I tell her 'it's complicated' but 'it should all work out'. I'm so convincing that I almost believe myself. In actual fact, the vice is tightening ruthlessly now. My immune system is dangerously weak and the transfusions are becoming less and less effective.

I'm fighting this illness that I barely understand like a lion. But right now, I'm actually a pussycat in oversized pyjamas who's fooling no one, not even himself.

The film publicist calls me. The schedule is filling up and I've no idea what to say. If I start turning down interviews now,

---

* A TV show on the channel Canal+ where, on 5 November 2007, the dream of making a film began to turn into reality after I met producer Luc Besson. I'm due to make another appearance on the show, alongside Luc, to coincide with the film's release.

they'll cancel everything. I carry on saying yes to the important ones, gambling on being granted a reprieve by the medical team.

I return to the hospital for the latest blood test, which could be decisive. Then I'm straight into an interview with my co-director, who ends up shattering a plastic stool and winding up splat on the floor at the feet of a stunned journalist. I can only thank him for the bout of laughing apnoea that ensues.

I'm getting a nosebleed. Bathroom, quick sharp. I just about manage to stem the flow with Coalgan. I check I haven't missed any calls from the hospital. The interview comes to an end. Dame Oclès is twirling her sabre and singing a lullaby. The sword slices through the air like helicopter blades. I block out my anxiety with a packet of nuts and a lengthy phone call to my sister. She is an excellent anti-terror defence system. The call-waiting tone interrupts me. I look at the phone: it's my haematologist's number.

'Hello, Monsieur Malzieu. So . . . Today's results are more or less stable and given that the next two weeks are crucial for you, we've decided to bring you in on 6 February.'

'Oh, thank you! Thank you so much.'

'I'm happy for you . . . But do be careful and if you get a temperature or anything at all, please call us.'

'Absolutely. Thanks so much.'

I pump my fist, John McEnroe after a winning volley. Barring catastrophe, I'm going to see this through. I must forget about the hospital and its ghosts as best I can until 5 February. I've got two weeks to negotiate a minefield. The countdown has started.

A grand *Grand Journal*

31 January 2014

The preview is in three days, the film's release in five and my entrance into the sterile bubble in six. Here I am on *Le Grand Journal*. She may not be here any more, but it's my mum's birthday. If only she could see me on the telly . . . I can just imagine the face she'd make. I'm called into make-up; it takes longer than usual now I've turned into a vampire. I'm bricking it. Adrenaline overdose. I'm wondering how I'm going to string a sentence together without stammering.

They come and get us. The speed-walk to the studio floor puffs me out.

I shift around on my plastic stool. To my left is Luc Besson; in my right jacket pocket is a sterile compress; in the middle, balancing my febrile emotions, I'm wearing a tie knotted by Rosy. Yesterday, I was in a grump because I was stressed and an invisible assassin was playing around with a screwdriver in my stomach. Rosy, meanwhile, was online learning how to tie a tie. She knotted three for me so that I had a choice. The one I picked is helping me keep my balance, stay centred. I'm trying not to think about having one of the greatest-ever French directors – who lent me his support for six years and produced my film – on one side and, on the other, a sterile compress to stop a possible nosebleed caused by an unfathomable whirlwind of an illness. The studio floor feels huge; I feel even smaller than usual.

I'm gripping my harmonica to channel my adrenaline. I'm a bit all over the place. Everything's happening so fast. Questions from the presenter Antoine de Caunes, a song from Étienne Daho, a pre-recorded interview with Olivia,* so tender it breaks my heart. I see myself three years ago, waiting for her in the apartment we shared. I'd shaved specially, I remember. I helped carry her enormous case filled with dresses – and anvils, judging by the weight – up four and a half flights of stairs. She had a funny look on her face but I couldn't help feeling overjoyed. When we got upstairs, she left me. I haven't had a proper shave since.

Everyone claps Olivia and now I've got to say something.

Not easy to smile when you're clenching your teeth, especially if you're a vampire. My heart is palpitating against the compress as I talk about the clockwork transplant in *Jack and the Cuckoo-Clock Heart*.

I'm frightened of bleeding and crying and stuttering my way through this emotional car crash. Dame Oclès is sitting next to Antoine de Caunes. I'm not looking at her. So I can focus on the questions he's asking.

The atmosphere's light, the rhythm pacy and I'm trying to

---

* A *grande chanteuse* of small stature who starred in my film, and my life until 2011.

keep afloat. Make them think that I'm cool with this – and me for that matter: 'Oh you know, just swung by *Le Grand Journal* to have a chat about my film.' But really, my head is like Mount Etna. It's hot on stage. My nose does bleed a bit, but only in the ad break. No one notices. They all seem pretty happy, so I am too.

The night before the morning after

1 February 2014

It's the last Saturday before I go into hospital. In five days, I'll be given a serum that could cure me . . . or kill me. In my latest hospital report, which I'm finding harder and harder to read, it says 'severe aplastic anaemia'. I flirted with danger a moment ago by skating a few metres to buy a paper. I had a little taste of sky, clouds yellowing in the late afternoon. I could have been inside an old photograph taken in my not-so-distant past. I've got an urge to talk to people I don't know. To improvise, the way you do in a far-flung country, when the excitement of discovery makes you drop your guard. A little old man is watching an English football match by himself in a bar. He's got a long white beard, Walt Whitman-style. I feel like having a chat with him, eating peanuts, drinking a mojito. My *quartier* has become an exotic land now I'm spending my waking hours shut away in my *apartshop*.*

★

---

* A magical place populated by skateboards, vinyl and surprises that is both my apartment and my creative workshop.

The final sprint. The preview. Dashing here and there for interviews. Family, friends, the band, the film people, Rosy and
Olivia. A new cocktail of contrasting feelings. It's important
to focus on the joy. I get a sudden urge to jump up on the seats
with my harmonica. I scramble over one and come face to face
with my haematologist, who has swapped her kind voice for
a worried look.

The screening is under way. I know every shot of the film
by heart, but I could be watching it for the last time. I find a
way of shedding tears on the inside. I want the screening to
last for ever. Not to have to leave the cinema, not say goodbye
to everyone at the end, not go into intensive care in four days.
The hourglass has nearly run dry. In the final scene, time stands
still. I will it to happen for real. And it does, if only for a few
seconds. I'm crying snowflakes. People think it's in the film, but
really it's me. Here and now. Surrounded by a friendly crowd,
but more alone in the world than Robinson Crusoe. Children
ask me to sign their posters; they're coughing, sneezing, smiling
and demanding photos and kisses. I don't know a sweeter way
of putting my life in danger.

Film versus hospital

5 February 2014

The countdown is accelerating. Here I am on the day of the release, the day before I'm due to go back inside. Film versus hospital. Putting on my favourite suit for the last time, before it's replaced with pyjamas. Flying visits to four different cinema screens to introduce the film with a blast on my harmonica. The joy of Malzieu's last stand. Giving Dame Oclès the finger one final time.

Night falls. Raucous crows evaporate into the twilight. It isn't the coldest day on earth, but it's not far off. The film guys head to a restaurant to celebrate and wait for news of the box-office figures for the opening day. These will determine the lifespan and success of the film. Six years of work and dreams reduced to a roll of the dice. I knock back my pills with champagne. Fuck(ed) it. Midnight. My carriage turns into a pumpkin. Cinders is scared shitless. My powers are dwindling. I'm dissolving in thin air. The first box-office figures come in. The film's blood count. And what does it do to me? Everything. I feel everything. From a speck of disappointment to joy, from pity for my vampire self to fear, it all goes through me, piercing me to the quick as if I'm caught in a Wild West gunfight with myself.

Two o'clock in the morning. The restaurant is emptying. Someone's turned off the music; time to go home. So I go home. I would have loved to carry on dancing, albeit slowly. Everyone says their drawn-out goodbyes. The taxi seems to morph into a high-class ambulance. I want to tell the driver to put his foot down all the way to the ocean for breakfast on the waterfront. Wanted: vampire on the run from medical authorities, sought up and down the coast. Description: very white, very small, skateboards in slow motion.

I open the door to my apartment like a melancholic burglar. It's gone three in the morning. Not long before today becomes tomorrow morning. Rosy wakes up; we whisper reassuring jokes to each other. Then it's time for seriously cosy snuggling-down.

Except sleep doesn't come. Naked, I go to the fridge to get a Coke. Down it ice-cold, blub bubbles. Snack at four in the morning, watching the stars twinkling in the mist like a failed firework display. Watching Rosy sleep, her breasts rising to the surface of the duvet like îles *flottantes*. Seeing daybreak rub out the moon with a cloud-shaped eraser. Taking a double dose of sleeping pills and going under at last.

Into the bubble

6 February 2014

This time there's no champagne or harmonica to push back the deadline. While the taxi's taking me to Hôpital Cochin, some of the film guys are flying off for a screening at the Berlin Film Festival. I've made the journey from home to the hospital so many times the car seems to be on autopilot.

The Achard building, fourth floor. I know this nuclear reactor so well, peopled by friendly ghosts who smile behind their masks. Rosy helps me carry my stuff; we're off on our hols to hell. We'll be separated. For the duration of my stay in hospital we won't be able to kiss or touch. We have to keep each other at eye-beam length. Mask, surgical cap, blue overall – blue all over. I am officially admitted to the sterile room.

I'm not allowed anything here, except rest. I've been put into an aquarium minus the water. Vacuum-packed exotic fish come to take my temperature. Two large rectangular windows offer a fantastic vista over the *quartier* of Saint-Germain. The rest is just linoleum, plastic cupboards and a remote-controlled bed. And, thank goodness, an exercise bike.

I place my rock-star outfit in a hospital bag that's identical to the one I was handed after my mother died, and pull on the medical prisoner's uniform: paper pyjamas. Suddenly, I feel very old indeed.

Rosy leaves for work. As soon as she's gone, Dame Oclès takes her place.

A memory comes back to me of a day with my mother in a similar sort of hospital room to this. She was so tired that she slept virtually the whole time. The situation was giving me a stomach ache. When my mum woke up, she said to me:

'You don't look right. What's the matter?'

'Oh . . . nothing, don't worry.'

'Come on, you and I go way back,' she said with a wink. 'What's up?'

'A slight tummy ache, but it's fine . . .'

She called a nurse and asked her to give me an antispasmodic. I was embarrassed at the time, but the tablet quickly made me better. Mum fell back to sleep. A few days later, she was gone.

Since my diagnosis, I've been trying to protect my dad and my sister from making comparisons with my mum's illness. To protect myself, too. But the differences in our conditions can't stop the echo of past anxieties resounding loudly. In this room full of emptiness, it's deafening.

A medical team shows up all of a sudden, dragging me from my sombre thoughts. 'We're going to fit you with a central venous catheter, to save you having jabs every day for transfusions and medication. From now on, everything will come through this. A lot more comfortable for you.'

Three anaesthetizing sting-burns later, the senior registrar is tinkering with a few things around heart level. They're wiring me up. Sew, stitch, prick. I could be in my film. I try making a few jokes to the doctors and they smile out of kindness. We all battle anxiety in our own ways.

I'm left with a dressing the size of a nappy strapped over my lung and a plastic tube attached to a huge white machine. 'It's a syringe pump,' a nurse explains. 'To regulate the flow of your medication.' It sounds like a percolator, but it doesn't make coffee. Little lights flash and when an air bubble gets trapped, it makes a hell of a racket. This robot will be my room-mate day and night. Above my bed, there's a sort of giant waffle iron. They call it 'the flux machine' and it filters air, a bit like water is filtered in an aquarium. It's an anti-germ shield to replace my immune system while I'm in hospital. 'A fortnight, three weeks, sometimes more,' the haematologist-with-the-kind-voice tells me.

I've been here two hours and yesterday already seems to belong to a distant past. I climb on to the bike provided and pedal, looking out of the window. The wire attached to the catheter catches under one of the pedals and the sharp pain reminds me how much of a hostage I am to this machine. Dame Oclès settles down on my bed smoking a thin cigarette. She's spewing out charcoal smoke that crawls across the ceiling over my head. I keep pedalling.

Night draws in and repaints the walls of the room. It's time to turn on the neon strips in the bathroom. The evening meal arrives with its smells from the canteen of death. Lucky I ate those chocolate biscuits last night because it's back to aluminium trays of overcooked white rice.

I haven't gone to pieces all day.

Then someone tells me that the man who looked distinguished in tracksuit bottoms, who sounded like a songless Leonard Cohen, has stopped speaking for good.

Dame Oclès hogs the bed. Her skin is snake-cold. She sleeps with her sword. The base of the bed is a blow-up mattress, like the sort you lark about on at the swimming pool, covered in a sheet. Very good for a bad back! 'Easier to wash if there's any bleeding,' someone explains. I try reading to take my mind off things, but I can't concentrate. In a sterile room, the minute you dream, your eyes start leaking. Particularly if you don't know when or how you're getting out.

My only possible act of resistance is writing. This crisis is germinating seeds of ideas for books. I water them all and do my best to tell myself that I'm going to find my magic bean and burst through the hospital ceiling.

The nymphirmary

I've done half an hour cycling on the spot, looking out of the window, with the sounds of Ennio Morricone blaring from my iPhone. Because your surroundings aren't moving, you have to find the motivation to keep going in the depths of your brain. Then I washed my mane over a basin with cotton gloves on. The sterile soap that doubles as shampoo is about as effective as dregs of flat Coke. It takes me an age to dry myself. 'À la guerre *comme à la guerre*,' my mum used to say. In times of war we have to make do.

A nurse comes into my room with an armful of freaky gifts. 'All right, Monsieur Malzieu? We can start the ALG.' The pouches of anti-lymphocyte globulin look like enormous packets of sweets. A blood-pressure monitor is fitted to my arm. I'll be wearing it throughout the treatment. This latest gizmo will take my blood pressure automatically every ten minutes for twelve hours. My temperature will be taken every two hours and I'm not allowed to draw the curtain around the bed. 'I need to be able to see you're breathing,' the nurse tells me.

Next it's the turn of the junior doctor and a little army of masked haematologists. 'You might start shivering and get a temperature. Don't hesitate to call if you don't feel well. The treatment will take four days. Keep your spirits up. It'll be fine.'

The anti-lymphocyte globulin is flowing in my veins. I'm milk on the stove now. To be supervised (though there's nothing 'super' about it). To prevent the treatment causing inflammation, I'm also put on a high dose of corticosteroids. Usefully, this medication also sets my nerves on edge. I'm both extremely tired and unable to sleep.

My finger is gripped by a little plastic pincer that monitors my oxygen saturation and heart rate. When I turn over to get my phone, it unclips and goes off like a fire alarm. The blood-pressure monitor tests my patience every ten minutes. A foghorn sounds and the armband inflates around my bicep. Every time I stand up, I get the tubes from the drips, the blood-pressure monitor and the heart monitor tangled up. The same thing happens on stage with the microphone and guitar cables. Oh Dionysos, my electric tribe, I've embarked on a pretty icy musical slam session. Keep playing: I don't know how yet, but I'll be back!

I feel like I'm in *House*, though I've never watched an episode all the way through. Perhaps I should have. My body isn't mine any more. I'm being turned into a processed sausage.

In barely two hours, the recumbent rodeo ride has done me in. A stallion of a migraine is galloping between my temples, stamping on my sinuses. As advertised, a legion of shivers is buffeting my shoulder blades. I've got to call a nurse.

I turn over to reach for the remote control 'help' button and knock it off the bed. I'm not supposed to pick up anything that touches the floor; someone's going to have to disinfect it for me. I try to stand up to press the button with my flip-flops, and inadvertently pull on the wire attached to the pincer monitoring my heart. Unplugged, the machine starts ringing out like an alarm clock set to rouse a whole town. I'm stamping all over the remote but the button stays unpressed. An air bubble gets trapped in my drip and the syringe pump starts to bleep as well. A symphony of alarm sirens. I've got the sort of headache you get from a good piss-up, but minus the alcohol. Canada Dry without the Canada. The blood-pressure monitor starts up. That's handy, we needed a few bass notes. I'm going to break the fucking help button at this rate. Dame Oclès is having a ball. When the nurse comes in, I'm kicking the shit out of the remote.

'*Ooh là*, what's going's on here?'

'All the machines are going off and I dropped the remote.'

'You have to be careful standing up like that, you could fall over.'

I do a little dance move. The nurse's eyes smile and, under the mask, I guess her lips do too.

'You're a right one, you are!' she says, fiddling with the machines, turning off the alarms and disentangling the plastic knots.

She hooks me up to a bag of medication to relieve my headache, speaking in soothing tones all the while.

'I've wedged the remote in the drawer of your bedside table. Call if you need anything, won't you.'

'Thank you very much.'

Her kindness has calmed me. She's a nurse-nymph: she knows a thing or two about sensitivity. I felt a tiny bit like myself when I made her laugh.

War poetry

10 February 2014

I've been here four days. I've withstood the anti-lymphocyte globulin fairly well. Yesterday, it flowed in my veins until two in the morning and we moved straight on to a two-hour red cell transfusion. I had a little nocturnal siesta from four to six, and then we kicked off the new day with a blood test.

Only four days in and already the outside world is becoming an abstract notion. Often, in the darkest depths of night, a nurse glances through the venetian blind to 'check I'm breathing'.

I'm keeping this journal like a captain keeps his hands on the rudder of his disembowelled fishing boat. An oil lamp flickers between my knees. The waves smash into the bodies of sirens sleeping against the hull of my skiff. A storm rumbles silently at my window. The stars come away from their celestial placenta and settle on my bed one by one. 'Oh Captain! My Captain!' says Walt Whitman. I'll need to construct some new haemato-poetic weapons. A mental shield so powerful it could modify my biology. The heart and its armada of desires must set sail to relieve the body. War poetry.

I catch my reflection in the shaving mirror. My cheeks are now jowls. Oh the joys of cortisone; I'm transforming into a hamster. I could have turned into a bat like any other vampire but no, when you're a small redhead, you go more hamster.

Every day, Rosy crosses the city and comes to me to smile at eye-beam length. With her mask, cap and surgeon's gown, she's like a sealed packet of patisserie whose orange-blossom aroma eludes me even when it's being wafted under my nose. I wonder when I'll be able to touch her, just a light stroke. I don't know what it feels like any more, to feel her skin on mine. She laughs when I say I look like a hamster. 'You're very handsome,' she says. I know I'm not, but it's good to hear anyway.

When hope's batteries run out, she turns into a charger and powers up my spirit again. When she disappears back into the airlock, my mind's sparkle-machine splutters, convulses and then falls back to sleep. Loneliness blooms. The emptiness builds and builds until it could shatter the windows. Then come the hours when I ask myself why my body has turned against me. Why did my Mr Hyde bump off Dr Jekyll? Because I've got the diet of a five-year-old with a taste for whisky? Because I was too violent with myself on stage? When I smashed the microphone into my sternum did I wreck my bone marrow? Was the trigger mismanaged love, amorous indigestion? Or never knowing how to say no and drowning myself in stimulating work? What happened?

Because I keep colliding with draughts, I have these purplish-blue marks on my thorax. I look like a red and white leopard . . . with extra white.

Dame Oclès holds out her sword, handle towards me.

'Go on . . . You can destroy all these fucking machines with this. No more beep-beep, total silence . . . But watch out – with your platelet levels, if you cut yourself you'll do my job for me.'

I grab the sword. Anger has given me a boost of energy. I haven't felt rebellious adrenaline like this for ages. I get up and stride towards Dame Oclès. I'm going to cut her head off!

'Ah, my poor man . . . You can't kill me – you created me! Your own antibodies are destroying you, your blood's worthless. You should be at the Berlin Film Festival for the screening of your film right now. Oh, and you're going to miss New York, Los Angeles, Tahiti . . . Still, you'll be back for the second film, that's what people are telling you, right? Ah, bless . . . There won't be a second film. What was it you wanted to do next? Become a dad, wasn't it?'

She lets out a peel of laughter. I hurl the sword at her javelin-style. Dame Oclès catches the handle mid-flight. She raises it above her head and slowly moves towards me.

'And now . . .'

A rotund nurse comes into the room.

'Is something the matter, Monsieur Malzieu?'

'I'm bleeding a bit in my mouth . . .'

'Your red cells and platelets have arrived. We can start the transfusion. That'll make you feel better.'

'OK. Thank you.'

Dame Oclès recedes and sheathes her sword. The nurse does her best to fix the machine that won't stop bleeping. I'm learning not to hate these devices. She prepares the red blood cells. They sound like more sweet packets.

'What's your group?' she asks.

'Dionysos.'

'I mean what's your blood group.'

'Oh, yeah . . . O+.'

She changes my catheter dressing, which I mangled while sweating on the bike. I'm entitled to a 'free waxing'. That's the classic joke nurses come out with just before they rip off a dressing and take your hairs with it. This one has unquestionably good technique and makes the procedure as painless as possible.

'I'm not hurting you?'

'I know you're not,' I say.

'It was a question,' she says, smiling.

'And mine was an answer.'

She has this little laugh that sounds exactly like laughter in the open air. Laughter in a bar or a cinema. A little white sparkle no bigger than a melted snowflake. It's soft and incongruous amid the bleeps from the machines.

Seeing the new blood enter my veins doesn't frighten me any more. I'm used to my vampire status. The transfusions tend to relax me these days. Dame Oclès is sitting on the end of my bed. I'm texting Rosy.

Rosy's eyes

14 February 2014

My beloved should be in *The Guinness Book of Records* as the hairstyle champion of the world. She defends her title every day by changing her hairdo just for her hospital visits, applies lipstick for the few seconds I'll see her through the slats of the blind. It's Fashion Week and a mini-model is lost in the corridors of a nuclear reactor. Every evening, when she goes, the emptiness gets heavier. If only I knew what date I was leaving hospital, I'd focus my energies on the magic of crossing off the days. But as things are, each day I spend here is just another day. I can only mark time with my bike, my daily wash, my injections and my writing.

So what if it's Valentine's Day? I can't even stroke Rosy's skin. Doubts stack up fast when you're confined in a sterile room with wires everywhere and a little plastic bracelet inscribed with your name and barcode. Your self-confidence takes a whack. Amorous desires become nebulous. Being ill makes you feel like a child and an old person at the same time. Deprived of a social life. Not allowed to work. This person's look or that person's tone of voice turns you into a fragile monster. And, more than anything, you start to frighten yourself. I'm always looking for something to make me laugh. Sometimes I don't find anything. A part of me got left behind in the plastic bag containing my clothes from before. My identity is adulterated; each day that passes makes the fight to stay myself more difficult. Because I'm a real vampire now. All that's left are the phone calls to my dad, my sister and a few friends. All that's left are Rosy's eyes.

Getting pissed on Diet Coke

20 February 2014

It's snowing outside the window, but my latest blood test seems to indicate that a white blood cell spring is in the air. Are the neutrophils budding under the sterile frost? I haven't crossed the threshold of this room – or even gone near it – for three weeks. But if these results are confirmed, in a matter of days they might consider letting me out into the corridor. Or letting me out, full stop. For that to happen, they have to be sure that the anaemia is no longer 'aplastic' – in other words that my immune system is sufficiently active to defend me from outside infection. Nothing is guaranteed.

'We have to be patient with this illness,' whispers my haematologist. She's come to encourage me and make sure I don't get too carried away. I think she's got me sussed. Two and a half blood cells and I think I'm ready to hit the ski slopes again.

Meanwhile, I've noticed my eye for pretty things is making a comeback. The magic spectacle of a nurse shaking her long hair loose from a paper cap is as common an occurrence as the aurora borealis over Montmartre. But sometimes, when they change shifts and the night nurses turn into morning nurses, I'm lucky enough to catch a glimpse of them removing their disguises. Their hair buns, apt to create the cone-shaped extra-terrestrial look, burst into life as if a spell has been broken. Rivers of hair flow in a vivacious spring tide. A sweet explosion beyond the blind.

Last night, one of them came in to check my vital signs: blood pressure, temperature and oxygen saturation. Like Sandra Bullock in *Gravity* just before her spacecraft is pulverized.

'Do you need anything, Monsieur Malzieu?'

'Yes . . . Kisses! I'm fed up with not having kisses.'

She laughed behind her mask. And tonight, she brought me a sheet of paper in a plastic wallet with the words 'Good night' and two red kisses on it. I'm picturing her and her colleague kissing the white paper, placing it in the wallet and disinfecting it. Then putting on their masks, caps and gowns to bring it to me. A really nice touch. Two mouths in heart-shaped unison to help my spirits sing. Laughter to calm the nerves. I don't know how many times I said thank you. It was like encores at the Paris Olympia.

'Do you need anything else, Monsieur Malzieu?'

'A *steak haché,* fries and a nice cold Coke . . .'

'The *steak haché* and the fries aren't going to happen, I'm afraid, but I'll see what I can do about the Coke.'

She returns with an actual can of Diet Coke. It's so fabulously unmedical. The typeface from the outside world, the flashes of chrome, the red steel . . . The satisfyingly familiar 'click' of the ring pull. Wetting my lips, feeling the bubbles sparkle on my tongue: it's better than a Bordeaux *grand cru*. The first mouthful of elixir and I'm transformed back into a human being. I down the whole can in one. I'm on the verge of fizzy tears; the bubbles prick my eyes. Joy . . . I didn't know getting pissed on Diet Coke could make you so happy.

Happy bird-day, big little sister

26 February 2014

Today is my big little sister's birthday. She's as worried as a mummy. She bravely hides her anxiety in the back of her throat, but sometimes I hear it slip past her vocal cords. I would have loved to surprise her by pitching up at her place with a skateboard under my arm.

Dad's coming tomorrow. I'm happy to be seeing him but horribly anxious about how he'll react. I'm scared he'll be upset by the arsenal of drips and by having to dress up like an astronaut to visit his little boy. When reality bites he must accept the unacceptable: his son has become a vampire. He may not get over it.

To escape the uniform of long-term illness, I'm wearing a 100 per cent-cotton white tee shirt that they agreed to bake like a cake by way of sterilization. I fell asleep this afternoon and mangled my catheter. I'm bleeding through my tee shirt, like I've taken a bullet to the shoulder. Perhaps I was dreaming of the Wild West and having a gunfight with myself. Unless I smashed the window and climbed on to the roof of the hospital like Tom

Cloudman?* No. Nothing so out-of-this-world unfortunately. I just fell asleep with too much weight on my left shoulder.

The registrar has patched me up with a few stitches and some disinfectant solution. When she speaks, the mask in front of her mouth creases like a paper-duck's beak. She's very considerate but all I can think about is the duck thing.

Rosy's been hit hard by the reality of our day-to-day existence, though I'm doing all I can to protect her. Where does this leave her dreams? Her own life beyond me? What hope is left? What does she think about when she leaves my hospital room and goes back to our apartment alone? Can she tame the ghost waiting for her in our bed?

The nurses carry around wardrobes full of emotions on their backs. Hope Transporters Ltd. Their weighty task: to diffuse a few scraps of light to the four corners of hell, where fallen angels raise a naked thumb to catch a lift. Dispensing hope is like dispensing medicine: they have to constantly adjust the dose. They are storks, mothers, nymphs, girls. I am so proud to know them, so grateful for what they do.

---

* Tom Cloudman is the hero of my third novel *Métamorphose en bord de ciel*. He's the worst stuntman in the world, a boy-man trapped in a hospital who will do whatever it takes to fly away.

Blood cell spring

27 February 2014

I was galloping on my stationary bicycle when my haematologist and her entourage came into the room. An old Folk Implosion* CD was sending electrifying waves to the depths of my brain muscles. Perhaps I didn't hear the knock at the door over the music. When I turned round there were unmasked faces all over the place, as if there had been a leak from the outside world. 'Your red blood cells are still improving. We're suspending isolation. If your white cells stabilize, you can go home in a few days.' Inner elation, similar to the day I managed to persuade a captain of the French army that I'd be better off honouring my record-label contract than doing military service. I wanted to throw myself to my knees like Yannick Noah when he won Roland-Garros in '83. But I restrained myself.

With their paper masks around their necks, they looked like a Tahitian welcoming party. What an honour: a procession of medical personnel come to transfuse me with smiles. Some of

---

* A great miniature-rock group, apostles of home-made playfulness.

them were delightfully unrecognizable without their disguises. I had an urge to hug them all; we're a football team that's just scored a goal in the World Cup.

It's the start of a new adventure. I ate from a real plate instead of a plastic tray. I left the room tugging my heavy machine behind me along the nuclear corridors. And I had a bloody shower. Diving into a lagoon shrouded in a fine multicoloured mist of liquid disinfectant. I thought of Rosy's kisses, Cokes in the fridge, my folk guitar and the plastic bag full of my clothes from before. I'll be able to dress up as me again.

A shave. No more Robinson Crusoe beard. With father on his way, a memory of my mother's distress rises to the surface.

Dad enters the bubble. It's hard seeing him here, with a surgical cap on his head. I'd like to tell him I can unplug myself, get dressed and go for a stroll around the block with him.

'I might be out of here in a few days.' That's the best I can do for the time being. It shakes me up to see him shaken up. He's overwhelmed behind his mask, though he's not showing it. I'm his son. I'm forty, but I'm still 'his little one'. Struck down with a serious illness. The order of things has been ravaged.

I lost my mother the day he lost his wife. His own mother died in childbirth, in the middle of the Second World War when he was four. He lost his sister before he met her. And now he must be father *and* mother for his ailing son. My sister meanwhile – his daughter – bears a mother's responsibilities on her shoulders. She bails out water from the breached familial vessel with warrior energy. My mother's ghost hovers. Right now, its presence is weighing heavy. Which is why it's important we talk about football. Tumble into a lighter world. Sport has been the cement in our father–son pact since childhood. To this day, we call each other for a debrief at half-time during important matches. On tour, ill, in love – or all three – it's an immutable ritual. Via football, he imbued me with passion and values that are pretty bloody useful at the moment. The surpassing of self, team spirit, panache. And how to lose without losing heart . . .

The ill wind

28 February 2014

Dad left and suddenly the wind inside the bubble changed direction, carrying off a whole load of buds from the blood cell spring. I needed more than 500 neutrophils in my blood to leave hospital. I had almost 1,000 two days ago, 650 yesterday and barely 300 today. In terms of infection risk, I'm back in the red zone. According to the haematologist-with-the-kind-voice, the number of blood cells may have risen artificially due to the corticosteroids, but they never stabilized.

Back to square one: my platelets will be recharged this afternoon, and my red blood cells too. It's all pretty fragile . . . With their eyes and siren voices, the nymph-nurses have come to lend me a helping hand. Demonically deluded, I'd been dreaming of waking up in boxer shorts at home, of lightly strumming my ukulele then going back to bed, free from wires. Snuggling my frozen feet against Rosy's calves. I saw myself chucking my pyjamas in the bin and going to see my film at the cinema. Breezing up to buy a ticket and munching popcorn during the trailers. Realizing a childhood dream that has been left hanging in the air. I already envisaged myself doing these things, so it's a bit of a stake-through-the-heart moment. That's what happens to sentimental vampires, I guess.

Even the bicycle gallop is to be rationed. Because my red cell count is too low, there's a shortage of oxygen in my blood: it gives me cramp all over. I don't much fancy picking up the phone to give people the bad news. My dad, my sister, Rosy, they were all so hopeful I was coming out . . . It's a Super Sunday defeat in the bubble-foot championship. I don't do goalless draws. I only know how to secure promotion or lose big-time. Today I lost a bit of me.

Dead leaf

1 March 2014

The drop in the white cell count is confirmed. I've only got 200 left. My immune system is shutting down. The nurses put their masks back on this morning. I was granted one final speedy shower.

So, I'm back on board the not so merry merry-go-round. Maximum observation once again, blood-pressure monitor around the arm every ten minutes and the machine for checking the heart. The house of cards I'm climbing with my bare hands has come tumbling down in a breath of wind.

> *Et je m'en vais*
> *Au vent mauvais*
> *Qui m'emporte*
> *Deçà, delà,*
> *Pareil à la*
> *Feuille morte.**

---

* Taken from 'Chanson d'automne' by Paul Verlaine in *Poèmes saturniens*. I have adapted a few verses for Dionysos's latest album *Vampire en pyjama*.

Off I go
When the ill wind blows
Carrying me
Here, there,
Like
A dead leaf.

Western in the rain

2 March 2014

Hope fucked me over, so anger has stepped in. I played the part of the well-behaved medical prisoner, I drank disgusting soup and I didn't bite anyone. I served my three-week sentence like a good boy, but I'm still here. They won't tell me the upshot of all this; perhaps no one really knows what it is.

How much more time must I do in prison? 'Maybe months,' a junior doctor tells me. How many months? What is this, life imprisonment by stealth? A death sentence? Reality is weighing so heavy I've lost my taste for dreaming. The imagination's magical remedies have failed.

The night stretches on. Rosy, my boxer with the mermaid's hair, is out for the count. She doesn't show it, but I know. That was a nasty blow, having got the apartment – and her head – ready for my return.

It's not a full moon, but the stars are flowing in my veins. I raise myself up out of my pre-coffin; a whoosh of air hits my lungs: the last hurrah. Dame Oclès is dancing and rubbing her icy serpent's skin against mine. Something in her electrifies me.

I climb back on the bike, put on my headphones to listen to the soundtrack from an old Western. I gallop, stationary. Drops of sweat bead on my forehead: anything that makes me feel alive is good for me. I want to get my body back again, even if it is booby-trapped. I gallop on, eyes fixed on the horizon. I've got an urge to unplug it all and flee. Bollocks to the transfusions. I'll stock up the old-fashioned way, from the necks of girls. I'll try not to sink my canines too deep.

Dame Oclès slides her sword on to the crown of my head.

'I'm not scared of you any more.'

'Perfect, so you're ready to die . . .'

I summon up a rusty old daydream: I cut the tube from the drip and put on my normal-man costume that's stowed away in the laminate wardrobe. Silently walk down the stairs in my socks. Retrace my steps through A&E and end up in the street. Sit down on the pavement and put on my shoes, breathing in the great night air. Careful not to tread on the plastic tube, mind. I cavort around on my own, hail a taxi that doesn't stop. Walk into a bar, order several portions of fries, all the Cokes imaginable and a bottle of whisky.

Maybe I'll bite, definitely kiss. Tell my story to an old man who doesn't give a fuck. Call my mates and arrange to meet up. Tell them lies all night, how I've been let out. Take off my jacket between two bouts of husky, hearty laughter and wait and see. The severed plastic tube goes 'ding' as it strikes the edge of a china plate. A-minor, I reckon. 'Have you escaped from hospital?' asks a pretty waitress, worried.

Run out of there in slow motion, breathless like an old goat. Hijack a taxi at a red light. Threaten the driver with a urine-filled water pistol: 'Take me home or I'll spray piss in your face.' The driver slams on the brakes outside a police station. Jump out of the car and roll across the tarmac. Geysers of blood spurting from my elbows. Catch the eye of a tipsy girl on the pavement: 'Hey, aren't you the lead singer from Mickey 3D?' Take aim at her with my water piss-tool. No strength to carjack another taxi, or even hail one. Feeling a wave of tears rising. Wanting to go back to the hospital. It's not so bad in this bed after all.

I nod off and slip into dreams of a Western in the rain.

The Return of the Jeudi, Vendredi, Samedi . . .

10 March 2014

After another week pedalling in the void on my stationary bicycle, the professor who heads up the department comes into my room to review things.

He explains that the white blood cell numbers aren't rising as fast at he had hoped, but that there is nevertheless an improvement. The cumulative effect of the anti-lymphocyte globulin and ciclosporin is not immediate and varies from case to case. If in four to six months I'm still a vampire relying on transfusions, they'll try a second anti-lymphocyte treatment. He talks of the transplant again. 'We'll reopen the search for a donor, but there's a 60 per cent chance that you won't need one. If your neutrophils stabilize, we should even be able to let you out in a few days' time.'

I've become super-superstitious. A scalded cat fears . . . not being able to have a warm shower any more. I can feel joy forming in the depths of my mind, but something in me refuses to let it show. Fear of falling back down again, even from a minimal height. I don't dare telephone my dad and my sister with the good news. But I do it all the same, and even though I insert plenty of flat notes, a melody of hope creeps in. Rosy's smile appears between the slats in the blind. Her lipstick is almost completely rubbed off by the mask, as if we'd kissed. Seeing her disappear down the shadowy corridor is a tiny bit less painful tonight. The nymph-nurses are working hard to mitigate energy-sapping. Nothing worries them. They come for a chat. Replace the antibiotic drip. Take my blood pressure. Make sure I'm not turning into a machine for thinking up superstitions. Inject some gentle reality.

Meanwhile, spring has come to flaunt its wares outside my window. The sun offers up her luminous *décolletage* on the other side of the glass; I can almost stroke it. I want to be dazzled until my retinas are singed. I'm a vampire who loves daylight because the memory of my human senses hasn't totally left me. Breathing in the smell of the wind, its taste of sweet chestnuts and dead leaves. Sticking a stethoscope in the clouds to listen to the rain being made. Eating winter's last snowfall straight from the sky. And what I dream of most: buying bread – eating the crusty end as I walk along – and newspapers.

In my own Star Wars, it really is the Return of the *Jeudi*. There's a chance I'm getting out tomorrow: Thursday. The neutrophils are stabilizing above 500. It's precariously balanced, yes, but it means I can leave this sterile room and its infernal machines, leave the hospital even, and go home at last.

One last nocturnal conversation with the nymph-nurses. A novel hope this: not wanting to see them ever again even though I love them. I'm a vampire of love. They are storks. Passers of fragile parcels. They accompany patients from the beginning to the end. They say, 'Of course we do, it's our job.' Spiders spinning cotton wool to soften the bubble's jagged edges, I'll never thank you enough.

Through the looking glass

13 March 2014

I've just spent five weeks confined in a sterile room.

I cried twice. When I found out the man who looked distinguished in tracksuit bottoms had died and when I was given permission to touch Rosy's hand. That warm, soft, miracle touch revived memories of buried sensations. Like hearing a song that reminds you of a happy time.

Today, I'm getting out! Robinson Crusoe's back in the Big Smoke.

Of course, Dame Oclès is coming home with me. I've only got a fifty-fifty chance of getting better and, whatever happens, there's a long way to go. I must report to the day clinic at least once a week. But even so, what freedom!

The joy of slipping on my socks, of feeling a tiny bit less short with my shoes on. My 'outdoor' coat. And the outfit's complete: I'm disguised as myself. I step over the threshold. Enter the decompression airlock. Decompress. And here I am, on the other side of the looking glass. Staring at my empty room through the little window with its famous blind. Crying like a garden sprinkler. Kissing Rosy in the space between two worlds, at the entrance to the room. Fairly astonished I can still master the art of kissing. Feeling invested with a new strength. More powerful and more fragile than ever.

Walking straight down the corridor and out of the intensive care unit. I've shrunk, everything's huge. I really am in *Alice in Wonderland*. And for once the White Rabbit – my sister – arrives on time! And slap bang in the middle of the Great Escape too. The lift is the rabbit hole leading to that extraordinary land – the ground floor! The little shop opposite the hospital that sells lousy croissants, lukewarm drinks and yesterday's papers . . . It's all extraordinary. The throbbing hive of the world: these people with no gowns, no masks . . .

Swallowing a ray of sunshine in the car park and sinking into the passenger seat of Rosy's funny little car. Crossing a jungle of honking horns. Getting stopped by the police because the number plate is twisted. Discovering the MOT is out of date. 'By rights, I should seize your vehicle,' says the officer, his voice full of moralistic glee that doesn't shift one iota even when we explain the context. Perhaps he's one of the Red Queen's soldiers. 'I see, but it's still the case that you haven't had your MOT done.' Rosy has kept her cool for five weeks, but now she gets angry. After a perfunctory lecture, the policeman lets us go.

Arriving back at the *apartshop*, which has been carefully prepared by Rosy to make my homecoming special. This is the kingdom of the White Queen. I feel like a privileged guest in my own home. There's an exercise bike, so I can still stretch my legs, and sweets everywhere – as if it's Christmas and Easter rolled into one. My guitar and ukulele are to hand and we've got new chairs. My sister starts making pancakes. Happy unbirthday to me! I'm Mad Hatter happy. I eat the puddings as a starter. Chocolate meringues, mint tea and the White Stripes. I forget to watch the Champions League, that's how happy I am to spend the evening as a spaghetti-sucking vampire with the two most important women in my life.

Then I slip into bed, with a human hot-water bottle pressed against my tummy. I rediscover the smells of washing powder and skin-to-skin chemistry. My whole body is waking up, the layer of frost gently cracking. I feel like I've been out of hospital for ages.

Extraordinary ordinary

14 March 2014

I have to familiarize myself with the extraordinary ordinary, while integrating my illness into daily life. Medication, dressings, trips to the hospital and taking all the precautions of an equatorial jungle explorer in my own bathroom. Learn to climb out of the nettle patch. Play at self-nursing with compresses and disinfectant. Freak out like a novice. There isn't a real nurse who appears at the press of a button: I've got to get used to being autonomous again.

Playing the guitar. Gingerly, so I don't get bitten by the strings. Doing the bicycle gallop in my *apartshop*. It's the same model as the hospital bike. Rosy found it, my dad assembled it. Nibbling at new experiences. Devouring Rosy's vanilla-yogurt skin. Walking on timorous eggshells. Off for an adventure in my *quartier* by night, wrapped up like a newborn. Not going inside anywhere so I avoid my mortal enemies: germs and viruses. Because my blood cells are still hovering around the red zone. Eating croissants. Listening to the wind in the street and the fizzy flux of engines, laughter and arguments.

Violent joy muted. Superstition. Fear of having to go back. They've just prised my body out of a plaster cast; it's liberated but fragile. I go on Facebook and I eat biscuits, but I'm still a vampire.

Happy funeral!

16 April 2014

I've been home more than a month. The blood cell levels are stable but not improving. I'm still relying on transfusions. The hunt for a potential donor continues. 'We're not there yet. This treatment can take up to six months to work. If things aren't getting any worse, it's a pretty good sign,' says my haematologist, who's become a sort of friend in a white coat.

But the bone marrow transplant idea is mentioned with increasing regularity. Every week, I wait for the blood test results like the Loto draw: there's a speck of hope but I don't really believe. Dad phones every day: 'And?' I'd love to give him some good news, but I don't have much, so we talk about this summer's World Cup in Brazil.

I'm to be confined to my apartment as much as possible, but prison conditions are thankfully more agreeable here. I can kiss, eat fried ravioli and sing along to the ukulele. The days are getting longer and I've started skateboarding again. It's the only infringement of the medical contract I allow myself. As long as I don't fall over, it's not dangerous. Surfing tarmac on Avenue

Daumesnil makes me feel like I'm back among the living. It's my little weekly challenge, going to have a blood transfusion on my skateboard. On the way home, I spend a bit of time at Shakespeare and Company, the bookshop recommended by Clémence, a *Poésie* expert on poetry.* Being surrounded by books comforts me; the place is an Ali Baba's cave for bookworms. A magical attic built inside a tree whose leaves are books. I have found a church where I can disperse some of my anxieties. Here, chilled out, I can venerate the gods I choose: Jack Kerouac, Roald Dahl, Richard Brautigan or Walt Whitman. I take a religious and playful pleasure in trying to read these authors in the original. The books don't make me feel like I'm ill and the people in the bookshop don't seem to be frightened of vampires who sit in the Poetry Room for ages and ages. This wondrous attic is run by a certain Sylvia Whitman. Same first name as my mother, same surname as one of my favourite apostles of hope. I like to think she's Walt's granddaughter. There's something angel-like about Sylvia – an angel who's really enjoying her new human condition. A sparkling and gentle intelligence. And everyone around her floats along in this relaxed humour. Even the dog looks like he's read Shakespeare, and the white cat you sometimes meet upstairs is so mysterious he's bound to write poetry.

The bookshop lies halfway between the hospital and the *apart-shop*. Here, I speak English with my southern-French accent. I explore each nook and cranny, play a few notes on the out-of-tune piano. The music of this foreign language transports me

---

* Clémence Poesy, an actor friend and neighbour. An expert in creative dynamite and source of great support to me in the writing of this book.

to another land. I buy books that my English isn't necessarily up to understanding; I'm becoming a blind man who insists on going to see the sea.

Today it's my birthday. Forty years old. I don't know who to dress up as. I've already been a Jedi, Spiderman, Clock Man and a very small giant. It's complicated being yourself, but now I do want to dress up as me. My friends have concocted a surprise for me. They're waiting for me at home. My dad's there, Rosy's smiling, there are pancakes, as ever, and musical instruments. We're singing and there's drumming on saucepans. It's a bit like an end-of-year tea party in a classroom of ten-year-olds. I have one of those really good times when I forget I'm ill. Until fatigue catches up with me. I've been guzzling Cokes, but the tempo's too fast. I'm 140 all of a sudden. I'm happy to see them all and touched by the kind thoughts, but I just really want to go to bed. I must be in haemoglobin freefall because my arms weigh a ton. I'd like my funeral to be like this: friends, good-looking girls and cakes. It's quite troubling to think that, apart from me, all the people here would probably be present at my funeral.

'Happy funeral . . . ' sings Dame Oclès, in a voice like Marilyn's.

'It's just a birthday . . .'

'Yes, but it's the last one, so make the most of it!'

Eggman Records

1 June 2014

The good weather's arrived, the World Cup's around the corner, I'm writing new songs and clinging on to my new-found oomph. But my blood cell count just won't rise. The treatment I received in February isn't working. The medical records now say: 'resistant aplastic anaemia'. The transfusions and gentle time in prison are keeping me alive, but the ghostly figure of the transplant is getting more lifelike by the day. Still no donor. Contrary to popular belief, you can't stay a vampire for ever. Receiving other people's blood is making my body stockpile too much iron. I must now inject myself in the stomach every evening and keep a little pouch on me for the following twelve hours: a portable transfusion. I've been a bit rusty lately, literally and figuratively; this prod-uct is supposed to remove excess iron brought about by the accumulation of blood transfusions. I have to wear the sort of bumbag I wouldn't be seen dead in on the slopes, not even when fluorescent eighties jumpsuits were all the rage. Sometimes, when I pull out the needle in the early hours of the morning, I start to bleed. The first time I panicked. Since then I've learned not to let it bother me.

Not getting depressed is a tricky business when you're condemned to going round and round in circles. I've installed a miniature projection suite in my bedroom. Quite a big screen, a few real cinema seats for my mates, popcorn and candyfloss makers. A dream service in your own home. Whatever it takes to keep Dame Oclès at bay. My collection of skateboards has been transformed into shelves, or skelves. The hedgehog and plastic squirrels are proudly displayed. I've also adopted the enormous teddy bear that was abandoned in the stairwell. I've hung him from the ceiling. The *apartshop* is starting to look like the inside of a Kinder Surprise. A cabinet of curiosities, where I'm the strangest exhibit. It amuses the nurse who comes to stick needles in me from time to time. When she gets out the medical equipment amidst toy pianos and assorted ukuleles, the contrast is pretty striking.

I have an insatiable lust for creativity: I face reality better when I keep it at a distance. It's become as vital to me as the blood transfusions. A daily sense of urgency is what keeps me from going under. It's impossible to look ahead. My life is governed by constraint, delay and vagueness. In response, I need spontaneity. I began by envisaging a TV show filmed from my *apartshop* or a blog, but I wanted something more physical, immediate and palpable.

Then: bingo . . . Not long ago, I bought myself a chair in the shape of a giant egg. I'd dreamt of getting this thing for years. It immediately became my writing refuge, the viewing platform over my imaginary worlds. The inside is red like the cinema seats, the outside white like a seventies lacquered table.

You could spend whole nights sleeping sitting down, it's that cosy. I write, sleep, read, sing, listen to music, kiss, and eat a considerable quantity of biscuits in it. I noticed that the sound quality inside the alcove is extraordinarily rich. So, I said to myself, we've got to record in this egg. Capture its particular sound and, just as importantly, its playfulness.

I give my imagination a grilling inside this egg; I shake it up and mix it with real life. I safeguard my capacity for wonder in it, protect it from the tsunamis of doubts flowing in my veins. It provides shelter for the dreams I've got left. Dreams that become reality when, with the inestimable help of Rosy and Don Diego 2000,* I decide to create the label Eggman Records. The idea: produce vinyl in the style of Polaroids. And not any old vinyl: the records will be white, like the egg's shell, with a red centre, like the upholstery. Home-made collectors' items.

I've always adored vinyl. Removing the record from its sleeve, then from its dust jacket, before placing it on the turntable. Delicately lowering the stylus into the groove. I love this little ritual; it implies a special rapport with the act of listening. My plan to withstand cataclysm: creative greed. 'We cook vinyl', that will be the motto of Eggman Records. We'll make records the same way we make food. The sessions will unfold like tea parties. Clémence Poesy or my haematologist-with-the-kind-voice; the cello or the ukulele – everyone in the same egg and the same boat. I love it already. It'll be artisanal. Party food and poetry. Readings accompanied by anything we can get our hands on: toy pianos, saucepans . . . Little transplants of joy!

---

* Friend and manager of Dionysos who has a severe case of poetic dyslexia. He inspired the song and short story entitled 'Don Diego 2000'.

Whatever happens, I want to fire-breathe one last shower of sparks before winter. I don't know what tomorrow will bring; I can't wait around until I'm able to record a new album with the group, write another book or — even less likely — make another film. So I'll keep this diary of a vampire in pyjamas night and day, and record songs and poems in my egg chair: the world's smallest known recording studio. This dream of instant output is a reaction to my house arrest. It's all about equipping myself for an adventure in my own home, going fishing for something spontaneous and something shared — everything I was forbidden in hospital. Journeying from home, journeying at home. Viva survival!

Giver

12 June 2014

I've just missed a call from my haematologist. I don't dare listen to her message straight away because she's phoning to tell me whether or not they've found a donor with compatible bone marrow. I've been waiting for this verdict for a long time. Every week at the day clinic I'm told, 'We'll know next week.' Today, we'll know for real. It's the search result from the worldwide register. I pour myself a small glass of Coke and open a packet of chocolate biscuits as a mock celebration. I settle down in the protective cocoon of my egg chair. Nothing bad can happen to me snuggled up in here. I play the pre-recorded songs on my toy piano, the music-box sound calms me down. I put my computer on my lap and activate the webcam so I can see the face I make if I'm told I've got a blood brother. We can add some special effects later: me with little blue birds whirling around over my head! A real-life Disney story.

Eventually, I press speaker on my phone and resolve to listen to the message: 'Hello, Monsieur Malzieu. We're coming up to four months since the ALG [the anti-lymphocyte globulin treatment I received in February]. Professor Peffault de Latour, whom you saw [the transplant specialist at Saint-Louis], advised waiting at least six months, which is still what we recommend, but we'd like to talk about what happens after that, because in the end, the options were a transplant, and given we're having trouble finding a donor as things stand . . .'

Trouble finding a donor? That means they haven't got one, right?

A cheery nursery rhyme from the toy piano fills the room. I carry on listening to the message: 'The other option is to do another course of ALG with a different product from the one you had. We were hoping to have another conversation with the transplant team about the possibility of donors . . . It would be good to fix another appointment with Professor Peffault because it's always best for a doctor to have the patient in the room to make an evaluation, see how things are with you . . . It'll help Doctor Peffault come to a decision, which won't necessarily be straightforward. [!] Please do call me back if you'd like me to clarify any of that. Let's fix something for next week – it's always best to talk in person . . . Anyway, I hope the transfusion went well. Speak soon . . . Bye.'

The jukebox continues its joyous recital. Digital birds are flying around my head.

Put simply, the ALG still isn't working and two months from now I'll need a transplant – but I haven't got a donor. The fallback solution: a second anti-lymphocyte globulin with only a 30 per cent success rate. Nothing for it but to pray that the first ALG starts working after all, or that someone who is compatible with me decides to sign up to the worldwide bone marrow register. A one-in-a-million chance, that's the official stat. And to make matters worse, I don't even know how to pray.

A sort of hazy stress engulfs me but I try to keep calm. The World Cup is starting in Brazil: this is no time to go to pieces. Eggman Records' first 45 is ready, the mix, the photos, the members club: everything is taking shape. Of course, there's always someone to pour cold water on your dreams: 'Vinyl? No one listens to vinyl any more' or 'Won't all this just tire you out?' They're right, basically. In fact, that's the problem: reason over passion.

Receiver

15 June 2014

So, I've just had a very humane science-fiction rendezvous with the professor who specializes in bone marrow transplants. As with the first consultation, he clearly explained what's at stake: since no entirely compatible donor has been found on the world-wide register, two 'solutions' are worth considering. He doesn't give me time to get weighed down by the bad news, but guides me directly to two new options. The first is for me to go ahead with a transplant from a donor who isn't completely compatible (nine-tenths compatible). In other words, a nut that's slightly too big or too small for my bone marrow's bolt. A transplant that's risky, but not impossible. The second involves transplant-ing blood from an umbilical cord into my body. A technique I've never heard talk of until now. Not surprisingly, since it's a relatively recent discovery.*

'The blood in the cord contains stem cells that are capable of

---

* The world's first cord-blood transplant took place at Hôpital Saint-Louis in 1988.

turning into bone marrow cells and promoting regrowth. The advantage: it's less restrictive in terms of compatibility between donor and recipient than a classic transplant. The disadvantage: instead of replacing a diseased tree with a new tree, we'd be sowing seeds in your bone marrow, so we'd need time for them to take. The aplasia lingers. We would have to allow for about two months in the sterile room and at least six months of being within easy reach of the hospital, because during this period you'll be very vulnerable. Clinically, of course, but also psychologically. It requires real resolve. That's why we only offer this treatment in cases where we can't find a perfect donor match. This technique is mainly used with children, but there's a good chance it will work on you given your small build. It's already been tried in eighteen cases of aplastic anaemia and worked in fifteen.'

'And the other three?'

'Died. But they presented with multiple conditions, were older or had been unwell for several years. The treatment is tough, but I haven't lost the plot or anything. I'm offering this because I know we can get your normal life back. Apart from your haematological problem, you're in good health, you're still young. That said, we'll be relying on you.'

'Meaning?'

'You're a musician, I believe.'

'Yes . . .'

'Well, you'll need to prepare yourself just like you do for a concert. Our job is to put things in place so that everything goes as smoothly as possible.'

'Like the crew?'

'Exactly. After that, well, we can't always predict what will happen with transplants – which is why you have to be ready. You'll find you build up extraordinary relationships with the medical staff at the unit. There'll be people on hand throughout. But the transplant will be teamwork. Without you, it won't work. The patients it didn't work for arrived at the unit with their heads bowed . . . You have to go for it! With the will to win. Try to think of this experience as an adventure. The goal is to save your life, so it's fairly important! Never forget, the bottom line is this: you have a real hope of making a recovery.'

I shook hands with my Jedi Master and left the hospital fascinated and frightened in equal measure. First it was my athlete's heart, which saved my life during the Dionysos video shoot, and now my diminutive size could open the door to a life-saving transplant technique they usually use on children. I'm a biological *passe-partout*. Perhaps, in the end, it was worth getting teased all those years . . . I'm going to pen an official account of my life's journey, to further medical research. I concentrate on the modest pride that affords me, rather than letting my thoughts slide towards more troubling places. A new countdown has started. I'm going to risk having my life saved by a new biological mother's umbilical cord.

And be born again. Which implies I have to die a bit too. Life is stranger than (science) fiction. I'll become a chimerical being, with blood eternally mixed. Just like Jack and his cuckoo-clock heart, nothing will ever be the same again.

First, I'll have to go back to the sterile room, to the self-incubator. The risk of complications during this period is high. I'll have to withstand chemotherapy and radiotherapy. I'll be dead tired (almost literally). I must be accepting and never give up. Rely on the nurse-storks for every little thing, and every big thing. They warned me: undergoing a transplant can cause yet more side effects.

But at the end of the tunnel is vibrant hope: the good fairy Normality.

Forward planning

I prepare myself like Rocky Balboa in the woods – but at home. With my ukulele in my egg chair. The summer slips by with the *faux* sweetness of a weekend break. I walk on water with friends (and a paddleboard). But a storm is rumbling on the horizon. Dame Oclès is keeping a watchful eye on me. This time, I really am going to have to confront her. Total body irradiation, my bone marrow destroyed by chemotherapy, a new dose of anti-lymphocyte globulin and then, let battle commence. Dame Oclès will attack when I'm at my weakest. I'll have to draw strength from deep down in my bones. Resist. From now on, I've got no choice: I must become a proper Jedi. I've got a few weeks left to finish my training. As I go head-to-head with Dame Oclès the temptation to go over to the dark side will be seriously seductive.

And yet, sometimes, I feel like everything's normal. Life is good for several minutes at a time. Especially during World Cup matches or when I read poetry. I'm carting around a dog-eared edition of Walt Whitman, as well as that apologia to bravery *Hagakure, The Book of the Samurai*. I used to read it on tour. Once, at the day clinic, I gave a copy to a brother-in-arms in the next bed. We both had drips stuck in our arms and were busy trying to comprehend the incomprehensible. He was quite old and kept making naughty jokes to his wife, who was sitting beside him, embarrassed. They were like two elderly teenagers. They swung from tenderness to bickering in a moment. After about two hours, the woman got up to stretch her legs in the corridor. He turned to me with a panicked look and said over and over again: 'It's war, being ill. War!' When his wife came back, he reverted to his former jolly self.

Another time, I crossed paths with a twenty-year-old girl with a wig. She was very beautiful, a princess with no eyebrows. Her parents were with her. She looked like her mother, who was crying. They were consoling each other with a hug in the corridor. The girl seemed to be floating above her difficulties. 'After this chemo session, I've just got one left and then it should be fine . . . That was the seventh and, you know what, that's enough.' Her bubbly girlish look was only thinly veiled with sadness. I was impressed by the way she managed to hold her course towards normality.

Then a bed was wheeled into the unit. The gentleman lying on it seemed so old, a fossil in pyjamas. There was an oxygen tube stuck up his nostrils and drips galore. A plastic carousel full of liquids was dangling above his bed. The nurses said hello to him as if he were in perfect health, and he responded with a little wave of the hand.

Later, you leave the hospital and get phone calls from people complaining about being tired, and suddenly you're tired of listening to them. Then you find yourself in a taxi with a driver who rages about municipal bikes, young people and traffic lights all in the same sentence. So, I'm always very happy to climb back inside my egg.

I'm starting to make a second Eggman record, though I haven't got the first one back from the pressers yet. I'm planning to make a third before the transplant. There will be mates, stories, tasty things to eat and white vinyl. That's all I've got to give. I feel like Father Christmas handing out half-finished presents at the height of summer for fear he'll be dead by the autumn.

Rosy, meanwhile, makes rose-petal light of it all. Illness doesn't take time off for weekends or holidays, it's twenty-four hours a day, seven days a week, but I think I can say, as calmly and powerfully as is possible, I am happy. I feel a new strength invading me beneath the tons of lead slowing me down.

That doesn't take any of the fear away. Thank goodness I'm frightened. Not being would be a sign of denial. It would be like not having stage fright before going on at the Paris Olympia, or having too much and staying frozen to the spot in the dressing room. You've got to go for it!

I have this ardent desire to go back over to the human side. I feel it rising from deep inside me. I am the vampire of love, my heart is beating, I live! I want to give my dad, my sister, my whole family, my friends and Rosy their smiles back. Live the life I'd planned for myself once the film was out, before I got the diagnosis.

I'd love to have time to slow down. I want there to be World Cups every day; football World Cups, yes, but also poetry World Cups. I'm planning to organize one in my egg chair.

People will climb inside the egg and be given a minute to do something poetic. Read, sing, improvise . . . Surprise us. The Poetry World Championship, just as we're donning summer gear and shunning our armour of coats and scarves. When the mouths of metro stations exhale human flowers garlanded with rosebuds, when everybody is so relaxed that even terrorism is passé. It will be Easter and Christmas every day, that's my forward planning.

I'm sewing seeds in readiness for my exile to the greenhouse. I write/compose frenetically, so things can continue to grow beneath the cellular winter frost I'll be experiencing. We're recording songs with Mike so that the band can keep up some momentum during my autumnal hibernation. This first step on the road to a new album is frightening and magical.

Am I making a posthumous one?

I have the creative appetite of a deranged ogre and it's growing, but so are my fatigue levels. Sometimes I even fall asleep in front of a World Cup match, one of the rare moments I allow myself to switch off.

Rearward planning

1 September 2014

We are D-Day minus thirty. A battery of examinations awaits me before the transplant. A chilling roll-call of tests to prepare my body for this latest nosedive into troubled waters. To evaluate my breathing capacity I'm asked to blow into a sort of tube linked up to a strange photocopier while wearing a nose clip like Jacques Mayol. An ebullient little nurse is directing operations. 'Blow-blow-blooooow! Hold your breath . . . And breeeeeathe! Veeeeery good! Again . . .' Half an hour of that. By the end I feel half-cut. I bump into dolphins in the corridors and mermaids on the stairs. Vomiting is a kind of dying.

A Walt Whitman lookalike is keeping me company in the scanner waiting room. I've got his book in my bag, along with some knackered harmonicas and *L'Équipe*. What the fuck is Walt Whitman doing in a CAT-scan waiting room, given he's been dead as a dodo since 26 March 1892? Do poet-ghosts still have check-ups to see if their bodies are in good working order? Does this reveal some melancholic hope? Walt Whitman gets up when his name is called. He disappears into the corridor. I wonder if the doctors know who they're dealing with.

'Monsieur Malzieu,' says a white coat. Now it's my turn. After the ghost, the vampire. Straight into a serious series of blood tests. A nurse arrives with a little plastic box filled with about twenty phials. You'd think it was lab-work in biology class. I've turned into a frog. I'm going to be examined minutely. If they keep looking, they're bound to find something else that's on the blink. Now, I've got to do all sorts of X-rays. I didn't know I had so many organs. I'm radiographed from all angles like a Hollywood star at Cannes. They're checking the module before lift-off. So far, so good.

It's been suggested I store my sperm in a bank. Total body irradiation could make me infertile. For the rest of my life I'd be firing blanks, like I'm in a Western for kids. If I want to be a father, I have to stock up for winter. This is highly disturbing, because in *Métamorphose en bord de ciel* my character* donates his sperm to the doctor he's fallen in love with. When he dies, she decides to inseminate herself with it.

So, I'm on my way to a new hospital to 'deposit a sample'. My seed will be cryopreserved in liquid nitrogen at -196°C, just like the cells of the umbilical cord they'll be using for my transplant.

I show my ID card and take a seat in the waiting room. There are four of us; I'm the youngest. The situation is so unbearably sad and joyful that I have the urge to joke about it. We're all there to try and save the child we don't yet have.

---

* Like me, Tom Cloudman, cited earlier, stores his sperm when he's confined to a sterile room. I wrote this story three years before my own diagnosis.

To contain my anxiety, I imagine a sperm-bank robbery carried out by a gang of widows. There are five of them, armed with pistols and iceboxes. They've put on their lipstick and done their hair because it's an extremely romantic mission. They're going to be mothers at last! This gang of widows holds up the biologists and makes off with an astronomical quantity of sperm, including mine. In a few years, perhaps I'll have illegitimate offspring buzzing about on skateboards under my window.

'Monsieur Malzieu?' I get to my feet and follow a nurse down a corridor that looks like all the others I still haven't got used to frequenting. I find myself in a room with the young lady. We both know I'm going to have a wank as soon as her back is turned and we only met a minute ago. She gives me a small receptacle and tells me I can watch a film on the TV or look at the magazines in the cupboard. 'When you've finished, put the lid on and then you can go.'

You'd think she was an air hostess explaining safety procedures. She's a model of neutrality. The door closes and the ball is in my court – as it were. I suppose this might be mildly more pleasurable than a bone marrow puncture.

My future children are not yet born, but they're already survivors. I may be a dead star but my frozen spermatozoa light up a potential future. If I die, I'll try to learn how to haunt my children without frightening them. I'll practise with Rosy. Even the very best vampire films don't have love scenes like that.

I go for a quick walk after leaving the hospital. I buy myself a few treats and pretend I'm back to normal. I go to a cashpoint, perfectly normal. Other people put money in their bank account, I put sperm in mine. But on the pavement, with my early morning croissant, I am exactly like them. A tall dark-haired woman with a determined look in her eye is walking up the street towards the hospital, hair blowing in the wind. She's very beautiful. The sound of her heels striking the tarmac is louder than the cars. Must be a member of the widow gang.

Mini-Westerns

13 September 2014

Another lurch of the rollercoaster: I've got a lung infection. So now's not the time to destroy my immune system. The transplant is postponed. I was all ready to go on stage; mentally, I'd put on my warrior costume. I was scared, but I was ready. Patience . . . I'm forever learning to go with the (contra)flow.

The appointment to fit the central venous catheter is going ahead as planned. I'm something of an expert now. To avoid injecting the thin veins in the arms too often, which would be dangerous given the aggressive products used in chemotherapy, I'm to be fitted with a needle beneath the skin at chest height, going into the vena cava. This is a large, wider vein, a sort of motorway to accommodate heavy medicinal traffic. I skate to the surgical unit. Destination: the waiting room of Hôpital Saint-Louis. 'Monsieur Malzieu, if you'd like to come with me.'

No masturbating this time, just three fat injections of lidocaine in the chest to anaesthetize me. People in masks, and a bright light shone in my eyes. Plastic gloves, then silence: I'm rigged up just as I was back in February in Hôpital Cochin. I leave the unit with a whopping new dressing sticking out of the top of my shirt. Then I go home the way I came, on my skateboard.

I quickly realize that I should think of these few unexpected free days as a gift. I don't know how yet, but I must get the most out of them.

I've just received the first Eggman record: *Mini-Westerns (with surprises)*. It's gorgeous, white and home-made. My heartbeat quickens as I place it on the turntable. It's a simple kind of joy, like eating your first cherry of the spring.

Time is speeding up. I'm going in for the transplant in three days. I spend a fabulous night recording the third Eggman record with friends. I'm having fun in my role of mini-producer. Sperm, songs, umbilical cord blood, records – I cultivate all sorts of funny things in my nursery.

I'm off to a midnight feast at the record shop Ground Zero to celebrate the release of our record. Rosy's made sure my last night of freedom goes off with a bang. We're a stone's throw from Hôpital Saint-Louis. Most people here don't know I'm a vampire, even though my eyes are starting to look very yellow. 'If your suit's blue, they don't have a clue!' The records sell like hot cakes and joy abounds. I let myself be carried along in the moment, even if black thoughts sometimes creep in, just as they did on my birthday. A lot of my friends are here and I'm wondering if this is the last time I'll ever see them. Even the haematologist-with-the-kind-voice has come. For the second time this year, I feel like I'm attending my own funeral. I'm terrified, although something palpitating deep inside makes me deny it.

I dash about a bit, don't eat much, drink a little. I'm dizzy, but I *shall* have fun at the ball. I didn't invite Dame Oclès. But she came anyway. She's smoking her thin cigarette, leaning against the record-shop window. I'm the only one who can see her, but she's spoiling the party.

'Can't you leave me alone, just for tonight?'

'No.'

'We'll have plenty of time to have it out in hospital. Go away!'

Dame Oclès shrugs her pretty shoulders and drags her majestic shadowy self further off down the street, pretending to take her leave.

It's a *Mini-Western* party here. Being surrounded by a crowd of people who think I'm healthy is galvanizing. Midnight comes and goes. I'm taking mini-doses of whisky and Coke through a straw as if each sip is a magic sweet. People go home with vinyl under their arms. There are no Kinder Surprises left and it's starting to get cold. I fear these station-platform goodbyes. I've got three *pétanque* balls stuck in my throat. Rosy and I go home. I swallow my *pétanque* balls.

D-Day minus one

13 October 2014

Tomorrow, I'm going in for the transplant. This time, there's no getting out of it. Time will stand still at the moment of truth. In the meantime, I must wind myself up like a cuckoo clock.

Dame Oclès follows me around like my shadow while I get my things ready. I need one last skate in my *quartier*, to feel the sun set on my back. I bump into the friendly newspaper seller and the waiters from Le Charlot. 'See you later,' they say cheerily.

I react as if to say 'of course'. Then I pick out a load of new books at the bookshop on the corner.

Eventually, Rosy and I go to bed with a terrible feeling: this could be the last time. Fighting off this idea is about as easy as avoiding mosquito bites on a summer's night by a lake. It's almost light when Rosy finally nods off. She's wrapped up under the duvet like a human meringue, stretching her little Betty Boop toes as gracefully as angels who have no idea that's what they are. I'm so tired my eyes are stinging, but I take the time to watch her sleep. Stroke her hair, her back, her bum. Searing the sensation on my memory.

D-Day

14 October 2014

I must have fallen asleep eventually because I've just woken up – so late that there's only a couple of hours before I go 'back inside'. I get up, feeling knocked about as if I were an old boxer. I look back at the vampire in pyjamas reflected in the mirror, with the yellowy tint to the skin that you get in old photographs. I have my last shower and let the water run for ages. I wash my hair several times, making the most of the fact I'm still allowed shampoo – and still have hair. I get dressed and the tension inside me is electric, as if I'm about to go on stage. I'm restless and determined in equal measure. The combined fatigue of anaemia and insomnia is offset by something new: rage. I'm hungry for a fight. I pace the room. Gearing myself up for the off.

We close the door to the apartment, but not before I've taken a photo of my egg chair. I already want to be back inside it. The lift breaks my heart. Rosy's eyes are bigger than usual. Our kisses resound like a countdown; they're almost painful. Knowing I'll have to wean myself off them, I begin to feel less like kissing.

At least this time I'm allowed my red keyboard, my ukulele and my folk guitar, as anti-melancholia weapons. I've half
moved out, my things are packed into Rosy's car, and we set off.
Except I'm going on my skateboard. On the day I was officially
told the transplant was going ahead, I decided I would skate
to the hospital. Wearing my Repettos and my red trousers, I
nibble at each chunk of tarmac as if it were frothy caviar. I do
up my laces at a pedestrian crossing and the smell of a bunch of
bikes-for-hire goes right through me. I slow down around Canal
Saint-Martin. The people I pass look at me quite normally; no
one suspects I'm a vampire.

Rapid-fire photography: reflections, bridges, barges, cats! I
capture everything that might be used as raw material, to be
kneaded creatively once I'm a prisoner.

The stone arms of Hôpital Saint-Louis cast their long shadows across this cruelly peaceful afternoon. I could still get out
of this. Go on the run. Now that I've mastered skatheting (the
art of skating with a central venous catheter), what's the worst
that could happen? Could *anything* be worse than chemotherapy,
radiotherapy and a bone marrow transplant?

It's still nice weather, I could hitch-skate my way around
France. I've got my blood-group card, a little transfusion here
and there and I'd be on my way. I'd never be bored with a
board. I'd taste all the alcohol on offer, hardly ever sleep and
speak every language there is – especially the ones I don't know.
I'd invent one of my own. I'd take photos, write on the back
and send them as postcards. I'd learn to make wooden toys. I'd
meet Father Christmas or, if I couldn't find him, I'd *be* Father
Christmas. I'd build myself a workshop on top of majestic
Mount Larrun, high up over the bay of Saint-Jean-de-Luz, and

ride down to the ocean on an old BMX bike to go surfing. I'd listen to music all day and play it all night.

I'd launch bouquets of fireworks from the chimney of my workshop, build a moving constellation over the roof and weave hammocks between the stars. In the garden would be silver swings and a miniature deep-pile football pitch. I'd keep talking squirrels, and my guard dogs would be giant hedgehogs. There would be a half-metre active volcano for cooking omelettes – because I'd have chickens too. The only chickens in the world that laid chocolate eggs. Yes! Rosy would be there, she'd have become a mini-model and scientist of repute. She'd give conferences on Loveology all over the world. When she got home, we would make babies by dancing. When they were grown up, we'd install a hot spring in the dining room so we could have a dip while watching films. The whole family and all our mates would visit our living amusement park . . .

Zero hour

14 October 2014

I look at my phone: it's 14:57. I've got three minutes to get to the bone marrow unit.

Unit *Trèfle 3*, Hôpital Saint-Louis. Block B, third floor. I know these corridors filled with cotton-wool women, the low ceilings more often engulfed in shadow than light. You enter an airlock by pressing a giant button with your elbow, to avoid touching it with your fingers. In the space between the two doors, there are a few notices bearing the logos of charities fighting leukaemia and a notice giving information about the Leonetti law: 'End-of-life rights for patients'. I decide not to read on – the title's more than enough for me. I'm stuck here with my skateboard under my right arm and my left hand in Rosy's. We're dressed up like we're going to a White Stripes concert. The second door opens; we enter the unit with its colourful corridors depicting kids' motifs from the eighties, designed to bring some cheer to children's days on the ward. Once, they cared for very little ones here. On the way in, there are drawings on the theme of *le trèfle* –

clover – contributed by patients and their families. There's even a Betty Boop!

We reach an area that looks like a cockpit. Glass screens, desks, computers. Here, people work in the subsoil of existence, in death's borderlands. They tuck ghosts up in bed and serve breakfast to vampires living on borrowed time.

The storks are back and they say hello to us through mask beaks. They're gentle, under-dramatic and considerate towards Rosy, the skateboard and me. Once again, it's a five-star hotel welcome, but in a Formula One paddock. No jacuzzi or sea view, but top-notch room service around the clock. People introduce themselves but without any sense of protocol. The humanity of the place comes out quickly and naturally. This layer of reassurance helps establish trust.

A protective mental anaesthetic kicks in. I'm less scared now than when I had to leave the *apartshop*. A carer as tall as he is kind leads us to the room that's going to become 'my room'. I already know the layout: I came here for a transfusion before a trip to Copenhagen to receive a film award. The rollercoaster didn't half get bumpy that day, spending a couple of hours in the place I was due to spend many, many more. But that day I kept my own clothes on and made a clean getaway on my skateboard before nightfall. This is altogether different. I know when I'm going in, but not when I'm coming out. Or what state I'll be in.

The tall carer wraps up my board in a hospital plastic bag. A gush of life's most vivid memories winds me. I stay calm. And breathe again. The nurse talks to me about skating and takes my mind off the plastic bag. I tell myself that I'll leave this hospital as I arrived: on my skateboard. Making playful plans soothes my anxiety.

While I'm still not attached to a drip, I can stroll about my room like a tourist visiting a famous prison. The airlock I soon won't be allowed to breach, the window, the new bike I must break in. I've got a fridge under the bedside table, a sink that passes for a shower and a cupboard that passes for a cupboard. The ceiling is low. You could try telling yourself it makes an appealing writing cabin, but really it's just a gloomy waiting room. The atmosphere is less nuclear power station than at Cochin, because this unit is older. It's a bit like a room in a university hall of residence, but with a curtain rail high up around the bed and the vestige of the curtain that, until recently, afforded the only isolation to patients admitted for a transplant. The syringe pumps are the same as the ones I had in February, but this time I'm allowed to wear trousers, socks and tee shirts. The bed has an armada of remote controls: to call the nurses, operate the light and raise or lower the mattress. Everything is done to make life as easy as possible for someone who can't really move any more.

A lot of things are taken from you when you're put in a sterile room. Liberty, intimacy, sometimes hair. But not having to wear the pyjamas of a tired convict all day long helps fight the feeling that you're no longer yourself. Objects, books and decor are permitted and even suggested. You get the impression they're used to long treatments and high stakes. They only do bone marrow transplants here. Nineteen rooms, nineteen patients, nineteen invisible neighbours, all in the same boat: all with the hope of being reborn.

★

This is it. I'm here. At the foot of the most arduous climbing wall of my life. The roulette wheel is spinning.

No sooner settled than I have to go for some X-rays. I'm almost happy to have time out from my room. I return just as it's getting dark, like any self-respecting vampire.

I know what happens next. Supper on a tray and Rosy disappears. I know the obligatory feeling of abandonment by heart. It's the return of Love under Cellophane.

Ignition

15 October 2014

I've just spent my first night at Saint-Louis. I've set up an outpost of resistance. Facing the window, which looks out on a small garden containing a solitary palm tree and a few bushes neatly clipped *à l'anglaise*, I lay out my red toy piano, the ukulele, the folk guitar and the computer I'm writing these words on. I'm woken at dawn. Me, the night owl . . . Straight after the 6am blood test, I drink a mint tea by the light of the syringe pumps and take the helm of an imaginary fishing boat. I know I won't receive any treatment until 8.30am. Alone to face the silence of a new day dawning. I'm learning a new trade: tempest taming. At around 9am, it's the Vampire Special for breakfast. Very plain biscuits and a second cup of tea.

9.30am: cycling. I've always loved to ad lib, yet here I am, running like clockwork. Our capacity to adapt is remarkable. You have to freedive deep inside yourself, but it's possible. My friends were worried: 'Ooof, you should take films, box sets, stuff to pass the time.' Perhaps they found it easier to allude to the risk of boredom than the risk of death. And I understand, because until now I've also tended to downplay it for family and friends. Hope's been a rare commodity this past year. I've been handing out more than I possess.

As was the case during my five weeks at Hôpital Cochin in February, I find I'm never bored. I read a bit, write a lot and spend the rest of the time trying to form a balanced view of my torments. And not always succeeding. Dame Oclès' omni-presence gives me the blues, but when I'm on form physically I manage to nurse the flame that has always illuminated me. The flame of frenzied joy that makes you adventurous and sparks journeys in your head. That helps you invent things and reinvent yourself. The frenzied joy that gives you the energy to found a poetical party, an electric tribe. That makes you climb on a bike and pedal, stationary, looking out of the window from inside a sterile room.

10am: I wash, i.e. try to shower in a sink. My experience in hospital the first time round helps me get to grips with this mode of survival. I am an explorer of sterile lands; I know the dangers in this jungle of emptiness because I've already crossed another one like it.

10.30am: housework. I don't want to be working or on the phone when someone comes to do my room. I try to make friends. We talk about Morocco, our favourite foods, hope. We tell each other stories, *our* stories, and another wonderful bond is forged, despite the masks, the gowns and the surgical caps.

11am: doctors' round. Professor, registrar and junior doctor. Quite a battalion of masked gowns in the room. I'm exam-ined and given the blood-test result that will determine the afternoon's transfusion schedule. I won't be having a blood transfusion today; this is the day we start the treatment. Fludarabine and Endoxan: two different chemotherapies to ensure the diseased bone marrow is totally destroyed. The first is generally tolerated well; the second, on the other hand, can have more troublesome side effects. We talk it through. 'Basically, don't hesitate to call us if something's wrong.'

The bond with the staff is quickly established. These are transplant specialists. Just like at Cochin, they're experts in sensitivity too. Whether they're cleaning the room, carrying out a transfusion or delivering a teatime snack, no one is ever on autopilot. Their ability to empathize is a fantastic cushion. I lay my anxieties down to sleep on it. Their emotional availability is total. I'm getting ever more attached to them and it's happening at double speed. They are my home now.

The first chemotherapy session has started; so has the countdown. Goodbye, squirrel hair! Destroy to restore. I play some tunes on the ukulele to avoid focusing on the first signs of nausea.

Rosy arrives, her eyes exploding out of the gap between her mask and her cap. She possesses immense reserves of joy – hidden in her fabulous bosom, I shouldn't wonder.

Irradiation

Five days have gone by and I'm standing up pretty well to the treatment. I have swollen up a bit with the strong doses of cortisone designed to stop the chemotherapy wrecking me completely. I'm starting to look like an ill hamster again, but it's OK. A flow of dreamy thoughts continues to irrigate reality. Dame Oclès is here, but she's being astonishingly discreet. I'm never sleepy at the right times and my appetite is far from ogre-like, but I'm cycling, I'm writing, I'm singing. I even made a little black and white video for a festival that awarded a prize to the film. The mass destruction of bone marrow will reach its height with the total irradiation of my ill little body. It means I get a little excursion. The queen-nurse leaves the hive of *Trèfle 3* to accompany me. She's the one I spoke to prior to being admitted to the unit. She was sweet and honest, and our conversation helped prepare me for what lay ahead.

I'm dressed up like an astronaut and the expedition from hospital to hospital gets under way. Journeying from one lunar base to the next, I watch a film of Paris flashing by in the ambulance window. I make the most of this extravaganza of cars, bridges and tarmac. I'm enjoying the ride, even if I am on my way to be gunned down by X-rays.

The ambulance slows down as it approaches the new hospital's austere buildings. I could write a book about the architecture of Parisian hospitals; the only trouble is I wouldn't really want to read it.

I remove my clothes for the irradiation. It's cold. The silence is deafening. You have to lie on your side on a metal bed. Without moving. Get shot noiselessly. Barely a few vibrations. Still not moving. Twenty minutes . . . I'm a slice of bread in a toaster. Waiting to pop up . . . Still haven't popped up. Just doing some breaststroke on the spot in a nuclear sea, to finish off the job of mass destruction.

Done. Root and branch surgery has been performed on my blood-cell tree. Since that was the part of me that was playing up, you could say I'm not ill any more. Just the small question of total reconstruction. I've been reset. I no longer have any bone marrow. My body no longer has an engine.

The transplant

21 October 2014

Today's the big day. Transplant day.

Today, I'm going to have seeds planted in my body in the hope they lodge themselves deep in my bones and make marrow for me.

Today, I'm going to become the son of a second biological mother. Blood taken from her umbilical cord and frozen at -196°C since 12 July 1999 is going to flow in my veins. Back then, I had long hair, was in love with a taller girl and had just spent a month in San Francisco recording an album with the band. I'd like to know what this mother was thinking when she agreed to donate her umbilical cord. Who could she be? A neighbour? An Indian? Björk? This woman might just be saving my life. I'd like to save someone's life one day.

My body is ready to receive brand-new cells from my donor. I've put on my Spiderman tee shirt. I would have gone for my concert-wear, but I didn't fancy wearing shoes and a tie in bed. I think back to Joann Sfar's phrase: I haven't a choice

– I've got to turn into a self-made superhero. This tee shirt is like war paint.

A nymph-nurse as kind and gentle as a specialist mum comes to attach little bags containing my future bone marrow on to the hook for liquid medication hanging above my bed. 'I'm here to give you the transplant,' she says, with the smile of someone who juggles diamonds for a living. Those famous bags contain a ticket that entitles me to board a flying saucer and travel back to the land of the living. To go from vampire to human status. To kiss without fear of being bitten by a germ. To run. Jump. Sleep. To be reborn.

The nurse adjusts the drip and checks everything's working. 'Off we go!' she whispers, in a way that's epic and gentle at the same time. I feel as if the blood's coming directly from her smile. I want to hold her in my arms, stop her leaving the room. A deep joy spreads through me with such intensity that I can feel tears coming, but I'm not going to blub in front of the nurse, not in my Spiderman tee shirt and everything.

I spend several long minutes staring at the bag as it empties. I feel like a sapling they're trying to plant on the moon. The plastic tube is my new umbilical cord. Hope is flowing in my veins. I can see it circulating drop by drop. I want this to work so much that I'm feeling better already.

The moment the bag runs dry is a bit magical. 'All done, it's gone in,' says the stork in the white coat and beak-mask. It's a new start. I feel it, I know it, I hope it's true. A calm excited hope. Tears flow without warning. I relax, but can't quite bring myself to open a drawer and stow the bags that contained the haemato-poetic stem cells. Like wrapping paper you can't bear to throw away because it's been suffused with its special contents. I read the label again. My new biological mother is called DUCB-03765. My new brother or sister was born on 12 July 1999. My anticipated date of rebirth: 21 October 2014.

The minutes that follow become sacred. Not in the religious sense of the term, although deep in the abyss I did sometimes want to pray/cry. I think of my mum . . . of Rosy, family, friends and even Walt Whitman. They have all fuelled my capacity to resist. They are my petrol, my gas and my electricity. Since the diagnosis I've been given two Bibles and they made me feel like I was in that old Fernandel film, when the doctor makes a face and they send the priest round to talk to the old fellow who's about to cop it. But I don't think you can just invent religious faith. I like believing, and I'm something of a professional dreamer, but I want to be able to choose what to believe in.

Dead

26 October 2014

It's transplant day plus five. I'm holding out pretty well against the side effects of radiation and chemo. It's not time to do the moonwalk just yet, but I'm adjusting to massive destruction fairly well.

This fine Sunday morning, I got up with a slight headache and the prospect of a croissant for breakfast. And suddenly: blackout. Did I fall over? No memory, no recollection of hitting the deck. Instead, the blackest hole I've ever been plunged into. The end.

A lifeless night lasting minutes, and now I've come to. I don't know how I managed it, but I'm back in bed. Survival instinct, probably. Time ceased to exist. I don't know what happened or why. A blank. Not the wisp of a memory. The only thing I can say with any certainty is that I lost consciousness and, judging from the state of my head, fell over – either that or someone came into the room and hit me with a baseball bat. I'm leaning towards the first scenario.

When I woke up, I felt like I'd been on the receiving end of a bare-knuckle uppercut from Mike Tyson. There was an awful burning sensation around my jaw and beneath my eyes. I got back out of bed to check in the mirror: left cheekbone caved in, chin like a cross between the Bogdanov brothers and Desperate Dan, an enormous bruise across the right side of my jaw and a shiner over my left eye.

I was a vampire; now I'm a zombie. At least the throbbing pain battering my skull reminds me I'm alive. I must have toppled into the sink and smashed my head. I call for the nurses. One comes in and dashes out again for backup.

'What happened?'

'I don't know.'

'Did you fall?'

'I don't remember. I got up. After that I can't remember anything. I don't even know how I got back into bed.'

A buzz of activity as more and more emergency tests are carried out. The nurses and doctors remain calm but they move quickly. Every minute counts. The hierarchical nature of the decision-making process is both reassuring and alarming. The medical crew are at the helm of the fishing boat but we're experiencing what's known as 'severe weather'.

A cold sensation flashes across my scalp.

'You're a toughie, aren't you?' says Dame Oclès, smiling.

'I do my best.'

'Ah, but you can't do a lot now. Not with my sword stuck in your head.'

A team of nurses comes into the room with a huge machine on a trolley. They stick metallic stickers all over my skin. I'm plugged into a small TV that displays curves in spasms: an electrocardiogram. I'm ET when his flower starts to wilt. The bit where he resembles a flour sack and the strange spacemen do tests on him. I'd like to escape on a flying bicycle but I have to make do with being wheeled across the hospital for a scan. The doctors talk in hushed tones. I haven't the strength to ask what's going on. Dame Oclès is tampering with my brain.

'Can I have my sword back? It's jammed in your skull . . . You're going to die now.'

A stabbing pain bores into my sinuses. I sense panic rising around me. I don't know how but I keep calm and concentrate on my breathing. I've been warned about this: there are dark times with a bone marrow transplant. 'You have to live day by day and gradually things will improve,' people said. Today I'm living second by second, in-breath, out-breath.

They take me back up to my room as quickly as they can. When you haven't got an immune system any more and they've stuffed you with ultra-precious baby cells, the risk of infection is severe.

No sooner am I back than someone comes to take me away again. A second scan is required because I've had a brain haemorrhage. It's one of the risks with aplasia. The platelet levels are too low, despite regular transfusions, so the possibility of bleeding increases. 'We have to check the size of the haematoma. If it's too developed, we'll transfer you to a specialist neurosurgery hospital straight away for an operation. They'll send miniature sandbags to the brain via the upper thigh, making a dam, effectively, to stop your brain being flooded with blood.'

They're worried I'll have a stroke. Especially because a high temperature increases the blood pressure. Mine is 39.2°C.

I won't let doubt or fear prowl around my mind. I can sense

them pacing the peripheries, trying to break through the barricade that my eyes and ears have erected, but I do my utmost to stay calm. Focused, as if I'm on stage and there's been a massive technical hitch. I listen to my breathing, the rhythmic accompaniment to every minute that passes without some new disaster striking. Dame Oclès tried to decapitate me, but she missed. I've just got a slight head wound.

A haemorrhage. My sister had one when she gave birth, my dad's mother had one when he lost her. They have to do an MRI scan to confirm the test results and determine whether an operation is required. I've no idea what time it is. The race continues. In mask, gown and surgical cap, I do the rounds of various hospital departments. I'm starting to recognize the ceilings from my horizontal travels.

MRI: the scanner is a strange tube where you listen to freaky unsynchronized electronic music while lying on your back wearing a sterilized American-football helmet. They're opening it on a Sunday just for me: I'm a special emergency case. No need to go via the waiting room. I haven't got Walt Whitman to keep me company, only Dame Oclès.

I'm injected with a contrast agent so they can see what's happening under my skull. I'm nauseous. Don't tell me I'm going to throw up in the nice clean machine they've switched on specially for me. That would be taking the piss.

I don't know why, but I tell myself that it's Sunday and in another life I could be happily watching football highlights on TV. Then I think about sampling the machine's impressive array of noises, but Charlotte Gainsbourg's already done that with Air. I'll never listen to that fantastic song in the same way again. They take me out of the machine. The hospital porter keeps sniffing, inches above my head. That's more stressful than the MRI's electronic jackhammer.

Rosy has arrived wearing her Zorro mask and there's nothing for her to do except worry more than usual. You wouldn't know it though. She's the most tender rock in the world; I don't know how she does it.

My catheter is blocked. Probably because of the iodine solution I've been injected with twice. Rosy has to leave the room. A swarm of nurses do their best to unblock it, pumping away with syringes between two electrocardiograms. From now on, they'll have to check my heart is standing up to all this. The little pipe designed to deliver the medication into my veins keeps splitting. It spurts everywhere. I've got hornets under my eyelids. I can't open them, I can't close them. My blood pressure and temperature are taken every ten minutes.

After an hour and a half of tinkering about with my veins and the machines, the nurses eventually manage to repair me. I return to the scanner: gown, mask, surgical cap and Repettos. 'That's a good look!' says the junior doctor. Specially with the Desperate Dan chin, a Popeye-style black eye and the prospect of losing my hair in the coming days. 'Resus have been warned. If there's a problem, they'll have space for you,' someone whispers. The results of the new angiogram will determine whether they go ahead with the sandbag operation.

Meanwhile, I can't seem to swallow anything except the air I'm breathing. Even drinking makes me nauseous. Once my catheter's repaired, they hydrate me via my veins. It feels like my head has actually exploded. And according to the MRI result, it has . . . Jackpot: a double fracture of the skull *and* a haemorrhage. A broken sinus (stop the fight, ref) and a broken

zygomatic, the bone that moves when you laugh. To be honest, I'm not using it much at the moment. I can't even open
my mouth. 'You caught yourself good and proper,' says the
professor. The world's worst stuntman strikes again. Leave this
body, Tom haematoma Cloudman!

Revival survival

27 October 2014

Endure. Suffer. Can't even enjoy Rosy's eyes. Falling asleep in a sea of sheets. Sweat. Shiver. Sweat. Shiver. Sweat. Shiver. Sometimes both at once. A feeling of having a burning ice cube where my brain should be. Getting up gingerly for fear of coming a cropper again. Changing tee shirts three times a night. Sleeping in a sweat-soaked bed. No sign of the fever going down. The machines beep. My mouth is dry. Being monitored every half-hour. Blood pressure. Temperature. Oxygen saturation. I've got too much of a headache to read, write, think.

The emotional cardiogram is Siberian. Platelet transfusions three times daily to make sure the haemorrhage doesn't get any worse. I'm a vampire consuming ever more cellular petrol.

My body might be clapped out, but it's fighting back: the bleeding has been reabsorbed; it was contained in the periphery of the brain. No sandbag op for the time being. As for the high temperature, that could actually be a sign the transplant has worked. Despite the pain from the skull fractures, and the fact

I'm simultaneously sleeping all of the time and not at all, I cling on to this piece of good news.

However, getting food on board is impossible. I'm a vomiting Etna. So, my meals arrive in the form of white liquid in a large plastic pouch. As if I'm being given a milk transfusion. I'm being overhydrated too, to make sure the chemotherapy doesn't make mincemeat of my kidneys. I'm pissing the whole time and I'm swelling up. Ten kilos of water in three days. I've got Yeti feet. Folds in my skin like a baby. A baby dinosaur. I have to convert my Repettos into Turkish slippers so I can get them on.

My temperature rules out all social interaction. Even when the drugs are doing their thing, it never goes below 38.5°C. Most of the time I shift between 39°C and 40°C.

Three days go by without any development whatsoever. I'm treading a fine line, even finer than I thought. The bed sheets swell in the wind. The current carries me out to open waters.

My boat needs bailing, my oars are bendy. For a tiller, they've given me remote-controlled morphine. I press the button to release a dose. It relaxes the mind muscles. You're basically replacing fog with fog, but the new one's soft like candyfloss. The effect doesn't last, just a few minutes' respite.

Tonight, an armada of woodpeckers have decided to peck my skull to smithereens. I press the morphine button over and over again. The movement of my arms against the sheets makes this roaring sound and the drip's percolator effect is Chinese torture. The crinkling of the drip-bags being removed from their paper packaging bores into my eardrums, as if someone is sandpapering inside my ears.

I'm a very old person in a Spiderman tee shirt. I don't sleep any more, I don't wake any more. Winter passes by my window. It's snowing in my room, but in my burning skull the snow won't melt. My vessel idles along with the current, drifting to obscure lands hitherto unknown to me. Here, you have to be a real hope expert to flush out so much as a particle of the stuff. The lifebuoys are punctured, but the whole crew is busily blowing them up again anyway. A whale of a headache slaps its tail against my temples. My forehead is frozen; it's on fire. I'm capsizing. The nurses arrive. In bed, the swell picks up again, my feet don't touch the bottom any more. I stay awake all night. The old flame inside me doesn't want to go out. It's sheer nerve now, nothing else left to carry on the fight. If I fall asleep this time, I feel like I'll never wake up.

Eggman

30 October 2014

I start finding hairs on my pillow. Then handfuls of hair.

So this is it, the big day. Cloudman is going to become Egg-man. With a lump in my throat, I let the healthcare assistant – already fast-tracked to fast friend – clipper my head. First touch of the razor, and the noise reverberates around my skull. What Kinder Surprise will my scalp have in store? What shape? Dents, no dents?

The symbolism of losing my redhead panache is not insignif-icant. It's the tip of the iceberg of my personality. The shearing stigmatizes me with the visible status of ill person. I can no longer hide behind my tight suit and my skateboard. I'm going to frighten people, like a real vampire. Ever since I've known it would come to this, my *amour-propre* has become withdrawn and strained. But, curiously, when the time comes, I'm relaxed, like a kind of Buddha-pudding covered in swelling and bruises. I'm going to age ten years in ten minutes but I'm serene. After the haemorrhage, the double fracture of the skull, the fever and the vomiting contest, I reckon I'm about ready for an army-style buzz cut.

The clippers fall silent, Operation Egghead is complete. My hair's all over the floor, the nurse is discreetly sweeping it up. There's a novel melancholic weirdness about seeing your hair tumbling into the bin.

It's time to have a look at the vampire in pyjamas in the mirror. You know what? It's OK. I can live with Eggman. A Kinder Surprise with freckles. I now look even more like an OAP child or a young Nosferatu. I've customized a new puffy-chinned look, a bald version of the younger Bogdanov brother. I'm intrigued to know what image will be reflected back at me by the kaleidoscopic mirror of love and desire . . .

Rosy's eyes don't move an iota. She graduates in Loveology with first-class honours. Thanks to her, the transition to billiard-ball bald goes better than anticipated.

New hope

Today, a new MRI scan confirms that the haemorrhage has been reabsorbed. I've been confined for three weeks but my baby steps seem to have got me heading in the right direction again. It's good not going backwards. Even if forward progress is in super-slow motion. Eating, speaking, finding my human feet again; that alone feels like a new life hatching. My face is still deformed, but the bruising's going down. The cortico-steroids are starting to work. I take advantage of the bright spells without a temperature to get back to the helm of my fishing boat by the window. Tea, ukulele, guitar, Spiderman tee shirt, egghead – full steam ahead. I sing and a nurse dances in the corridor, clapping her hands flamenco-style. It becomes a sort of funny ritual. I'm cycling again.

The first white blood cells showed up in my blood test this morning! A piece of good news to be handled with extreme caution. But something has shifted. The time machine might just be getting under way. I feel like a surfer who's been regurgitated by the ocean. I thought I'd died in the barrel waves. I saw Dame Oclès dressed as a siren beckoning me downwards. Today, I'm sprawled out on the beach, trying to get my breath back. Realizing what nearly happened to me.

This new hope must be eked out day by day. Milligram by milligram, again and again, like the drugs. That's the deal I made with the professor. He knows what I'm like. I'm so happy to make progress that I feel like reaching for my skateboard in the cupboard.

With each day that passes, my temperature drops and my white blood cell count rises. It's 4 November and I've already passed the 500PMN* mark: I no longer have aplastic anaemia. I'm cycling more and more and I've just finished a song composed entirely in my sterile room: 'Hospital Blues'. Every morning at 6am, I take up my post by the window. I am a happy hermit travelling inside his own head. Now it's less sore, I can go further for longer.

I'm allowed walks in the corridor from today. Yes, I'm dressed up like an astronaut but I *am* walking. By my standards, a lift is Space Mountain. The ground floor becomes the Champs-Élysées!

Rosy and I explore different floors of Hôpital Saint-Louis. We pace the corridors, slowly. A reflection of the illuminated Eiffel Tower sparkles in a window. We go past the room where the platelets are stored. All these little bags of blood from

---

* Polymorphonuclear neutrophils, the most important white blood cells for fighting off infection.

strangers who have temporarily kept me alive. United in ano-
nymity. Givers.

A nymph-nurse is collating the bags according to patients'
blood groups. She rocks them gently, the cells must keep moving or they'll die. Then she attaches them to a robot that's
programmed to rock on her behalf. I could stay and watch her
work for hours. I'm realizing just how complex the journey
is between the blood donor and the recipient, and how much
expertise is involved along the way. It's moving, becoming
aware of the process. Like clockwork sorcery. In a way, that's
exactly what it is.

Rodeo

5 November 2014

I've got my appetite back.

The rhythm of transfusions is slowing these days, but a bag of platelets is entering my bloodstream as I eat my pasta shells with Rosy.

I suddenly start shivering, as if someone's just turned down the central heating inside my body.

'Shouldn't you call someone?' she asks.

'No, no, it's fine.'

But in a few minutes the shivers turn to trembling. I can't control my fork any more. I'm involuntarily playing drums on my plate. I'm the Duracell Bunny. A pasta shell flies through the air. I try to wrestle control of my tray, and fail. The trembles change to spasms. It's not just my hands now; my whole body is possessed with a strange boogie.

'OK, I'm calling someone!'

My forehead is burning up and I'm freezing cold, like at the darkest hours of the transplant. Can you get an electric shock from pasta shells? If anyone wants to do a remake of *The Exorcist*, now would be a good time. I'm being shaken by another me coming from I don't know where.

A nymph-nurse arrives and takes my temperature: 39.4°C. It was 37.5°C a quarter of an hour ago. She calls the duty junior doctor immediately. I huddle under the covers and focus all my strength on getting my breath back. The spasms are machine-gunning me at such a rapid rate that I haven't got time to breathe. Rosy stays calm and watches my every move.

The doctor arrives. Temperature taken for the second time: 40.3°C.

'You're having a reaction to the platelets. Has this happened before?'

'Nn . . . nn . . . nnnno!'

I'm the world's first stuttering vampire. A substantial quantity of pasta shells is strewn across the floor and I'm still dancing 'the jerk' at double speed. The doctor unclips the near-empty bag of platelets and replaces it with corticosteroids.

'Don't worry, it will soon pass.'

I'm suffocating. Drowning in a lack of air. Temperature taken again: 40.6°C. I feel like someone's turned on a microwave in my head. This vampire's got sunstroke. Pulse: 180.

Still no sign of calming down. I thought we'd rounded Cape Horn with the haemorrhage and the fall, but a headwind seems to be dragging my fragile skiff back towards dark lands. I'm only thinking one thing: breathe. Rosy is statue-still. The rodeo ride is intensifying, the horse in me is untameable, he's breathing fire in the snow. I've never been this cold and this hot at the same time.

At last, the spasms start to reduce. A bit less violent and more spread out. I've been able to partially catch my breath. The storm is moving off, my temperature is dropping thanks to the cortisone . . . Half an hour later, I'm virtually back to normal. The pasta shells are cold, it's time for Rosy to go. Almost like nothing happened. Blue skies after the storm that nearly carried me off. I'm told the fit could have caused another haemorrhage.

I find myself alone with Dame Oclès. She's having a footballer's crisis of confidence. She's been all over me for a year and had two massive chances to kill off the game and me with it. It was one-on-one, I was down on the ground, she had the ball at her feet and somehow she missed. Now the match could go either way. I'm still in it. And for the first time, she's having doubts.

The land of the living

12 November 2014

I've been so much better these past few days that they're starting to remove some of the numerous wires connecting me to
machinery. A year ago this week, France qualified for the World
Cup in Brazil by the skin of their teeth and I found out I was
a vampire.

Everything's happening quickly, all of a sudden. Today, I was
brought a leaflet explaining rules to be observed when you leave
hospital. Leave! A dazzling word that I handle like a flame, both
for its ability to burn and to extinguish itself. I still fear Dame
Oclès. Every time it looks like she's fading, she comes back to
attack me at close quarters. It seems crazy that after a year of
dense blackness, and so soon after my haemorrhagic rodeo, a
sliver of daylight is showing and I might be able to go home
at last, but they seem pretty sure of themselves . . . Don't get
carried away. Whatever you do, don't get carried away.

In my room, when the weather's bad, it's like night-time in
the middle of the afternoon. I'm still getting up before daybreak so I can see the first rays of sunlight bouncing off my

folk guitar and ukulele. I write this book and I work on songs for the new album.

Dionysus was twice born. First from Semele's womb, then from the thigh of Jupiter. The god salvaged him from the womb after Semele died in pregnancy, by slicing open his own leg and sewing the babe inside to complete its gestation. I've been twice born too. First from my mother's womb, then from the cells of a bio-mother fashioned by a haemato-poet. I don't really believe in gods but I do believe in Dionysos. Each syllable sings out to me. In my sterile room, I'm sent versions of my songs that members of the band have started to arrange. The prospect of singing with them again sends the sense of rebirth into overdrive. I'm coming!

It's raining good news: I may not be emerging from Jupiter's thigh, but I might emerge from hospital in two days. Just for the weekend, a sort of medical leave of absence. But if all the fragile elements stay in one piece, I'll only return to my lunar barracks for two days next week. Another rung on the ladder. It's not licence for hard-core partying, just hard-core hugging. A return to the cocoon of Eggman Records. The first big Kinder Surprise in the Forward Planning calendar. But first I've got to knock out a virus that has set up shop in my immune system's absence. Perhaps I should be worried, but the gust of euphoria about the possibility of leaving hospital has galvanized me.

This time, hope hasn't bamboozled me: I really am getting out today! With my guitar in a dustbin bag and my surgical mask and Spiderman hat sitting pretty, I find myself in the open air, contemplating rain with sunny joy. To prolong the suspense, it took us three quarters of an hour to find a taxi. Luckily a nurse-stork gave me a hand. She wanted to make sure her parcel was going to reach its destination.

I've hitchhiked across hell. I'm still there, but I'm sitting comfortably in a taxi now. The driver's yelling and honking his horn at red lights: what a glorious racket! Through the window, I watch my *quartier* unfold before my eyes. I'm not on my way to receive a blast of radiation; I'm on my way home. Seeing the wet tarmac twinkling in the headlights: back to the land of the living! Climbing out of the taxi, feeling the biting cold in my lungs: back to the land of the living! Mist up to my knees, feeling minuscule and giant-like at the same time. I've got an urge to run about. It's only a leave of absence, but I'm being reborn.

Crossing the street with my mask on, scaling the stairs. And opening the door I feared was shut for good. Indiana Jones and the Raiders of the Lost Apartshop. My egg chair is there. It's extraordinarily normal to find the cocoon as I left it. Rosy has done some gentle housework, I can tell. The nest is ready, the bed sheets smell of washing powder from another time.

I remove my guitar from its mortiferous sack, sit in my egg and play a few chords. Back in the land of the living! I'm still a vampire but I've got a new genetic identity; for the weekend at least, I'm becoming human again. The nurses aren't a mere press-of-a-button away any more. I haven't got a button. That's both pleasing and terrifying.

I refind my place in the heart of the home remarkably quickly. I raid the fridge, put a record on. I'm savouring every detail, from the noise of the creaky floorboard to the dimmer switch on the halogen lamp.

I climb back into my egg, overjoyed at the idea of snuggling down in my own shell. Crazy happy! Out of the window, a sunset disguised as the aurora borealis paints the sky. I take the silence's pulse, relish its amplitude and then go and fetch a Coke from the fridge.

I am the happiest of men. I have the urge to laugh and cry pretty much all the time . . . I'm at bit anxious without the nurses, but it's a well-balanced dose of anxiety. I'm savouring this new phase without downing whiskies or doing somer-saults or setting off on my skateboard world tour. Although such delightful ideas cross my mind, I stick to ukulele and ping-pong.

My little world hasn't collapsed, and nor have I. It would seem that Dame Oclès didn't follow me home; she must be waiting at the hospital.

At kiss o'clock, it's like someone reconnected the hot water in my heart. The vampire of love has his wish, the emotional electrocardiogram ripples. Because of the double skull fracture, my upper lip is still anaesthetized as if I've been to the dentist. It's a semi-kiss sensation but I receive the full force of the velvety wave. It doesn't take long to get reaccustomed to tenderness when you return from the battlefield. I'm so happy I don't even want to wash. When I do, it's party time in the shower: so good to be reunited with a gush of water.

I catch sight of my new reflection in the mirror. Still a vampire who needs the blood of other people, but in bald mode. Half Fantômas, half Moby. And in Rosy's arms, I feel like Benjamin Button at the end of the story. An old wrinkly newborn. Nosferatu in a navy jumper. I put on a bathrobe and instantly become a live-in Tibetan monk. I take some Polaroids. Instant photos, even botched ones, fill me with joy.

But the sweet interlude whizzes by in fast forward, and it's already time to return to the lunar base in the 10th *arrondissement*.

Chauffeur service

17 November 2014

Going back to hospital has the feel of going back to work at the factory. A dream-of-getting-better factory. To think that just a few Sundays ago I was being dragged from one scanner to the next with a chin like the Bogdanov brothers. It's only three weeks since the haemorrhage.

I have a classic taxi driver for the journey to the hospital. I get in the car. He gives me a look in the rear-view mirror. No hello.

'Hi, I'd like to go to Hôpital Saint-Louis, number 1 Avenue Claude-Vellefaux, please.'

'You feeling ill? What's that medicine you got?'

'It's disinfectant gel for hands, about as clean as you can get.'

He opens his windows fully. At 7.50am in November. So I explain that draughts are dangerous for me, that I've recently had a long stay in hospital. Freezing cold air makes me hedgehog prickly. His sneering tone isn't helping either. Anger's rising under my woolly hat. The driver insists I get out at Place de la République. He can't abide the smell of clean hands. I tell him again that I've just spent five weeks in a sterile room, it's not good for me to walk in the wind. But the more I talk about my health problems, the more aggressive he gets. He orders me to get out. I do as I'm told but call him a name and slam the door. Hard. He gets out of his car, runs to catch up with me, calls me *lots* of names and gives me a kick in the hip that I block with my arm. I almost fall over. He gets back in his car . . .

I head to the hospital on foot, wrap myself up as best I can, try to use the walk into the wind to dilute my anger. That bloke's stupidity takes my breath away. The experience jolts me back to feeling like an ill person again. Masked, and vulnerable to acts of aggression. To germs, to kicks, to cunts. I'm becoming intolerant of intolerance. In the sterile room, you can be an ex-ginger neo-baldie and wear Batman pyjamas that are too small for you, but you're still valued, respected and supported. I have to rehabilitate my mind for the outside world. Perhaps I'm not as ready as I thought I was. You question yourself when you feel fragile . . . What doesn't kill us makes us stronger. But it can damage us along the way.

At Hôpital Saint-Louis, the old-age child drags his imaginary fishing boat from storms to calmer waters. The medical crew keep check on the hull, the prow and the bulwark. Cape Horn and its sea monsters Chemo and X-ray are apparently behind me. A spring breeze is blowing. No looking back. Full steam ahead!

Made to measure

18 November 2014

The professor has just given me some good news. Firstly, the EBV virus seems to be under control. Secondly, the chimerism test (with a magical name) that determines the percentage of old and new cells in the blood, is '100 per cent umbilical cord', which means the transplant has taken.

It will take time to stabilize, but it's a crucial stage to have reached. It means my bone marrow is starting to produce new cells and my blood analysis is improving. The white blood cells are on the rise, the reds have stabilized and the platelets are dropping less quickly. There's still a risk of haemorrhage, a risk of infection too, but not so great that I have to be confined to a sterile room.

I want to throw my arms in the air as if our team has just scored in the final, but I restrain myself.

'The transplant you have just received is made to measure. With each blood test, we check everywhere and if there's the slightest warning sign, we take action. It's as complex as space shuttle ground control. Biologists you will never see are working on your blood analysis every day. And the treatment is finally tuned,' the professor tells me.

He's a passionate man. Possessed by what he does.

'But never forget, take one step at a time. It's barely a month since the transplant . . . You're ahead of the game, that's very good, but whatever you do, don't relax your efforts. You'll be leaving hospital, but stay vigilant – the slightest high temperature, a shiver or anything, and you're to come straight back.'

I'm learning to contain my joy, but I feel like I'm exploding with it. I so wanted to attempt the journey home on my skateboard, but I'm going to wait a bit for that. It would be a shame to get a little stone caught in the wheel and end up splat on the ground this close to the finishing line.

Resurrection

19 November 2014

Perhaps for the last time, I'm sitting at the helm of my stationary fishing boat. I'm leaving hospital this afternoon. ET go home. Umbilical Man is going back to his cocoon. I've swum across a river full of currents and crocodiles, and made it to the other side. I've got to relearn everything. But what a wonderful challenge that is.

This time, I collect my belongings from the little cupboard of death. Hats for the neo-baldie, old superhero tee shirts and the plastic bag with my skateboard in it. 'Demob', as they say.

I take Polaroids of people from the unit, who come and see me to say goodbye and wish me good luck. I've mixed feelings, just like at the end of my stay at Hôpital Cochin. Escape from Alcatraz mingled with sadness. I'm leaving this adoptive family, my bags packed with fragile hope. I'll be back to see them. I won't miss the hospital, but I will miss the people in it.

I have a last look round my room before closing the door with a frisson of fear. It's almost as destabilizing as when I left the *apartshop* to have the transplant. I've got this urge to take

171

photos. The nurses tell me that some patients need to forget their time in hospital; I need to remember mine. A duty of remembrance is imprinted deep in my bones.

I'm going to embark on a career as a poetician. Write a manifesto of dreams to share, and keep to. I want to live the best I can, out of respect to those who gave me their blood, their time, their bone marrow. I want to thank Walt Whitman and believe in Dionysos. I've been given a new chance. I want to press a button and send the magic lift on to someone else.

I pass through the gates of hell in slow motion. The wind could still change direction and whisk me back to the heart of the inferno. But today, I'm going home.

A gorgeous little female-shaped *pomme à la vanille* is waiting for me at home. I'm still handicapped in the kissing department, but these half-kisses are multiplying like stem cells.

The force awakens

24 November 2014

So here I am, in relaxed hospital mode, with a sprinkling of appointments throughout the week. Blood tests, examinations; they're still meticulously checking everything's working on board the space shuttle Recovery. The blood levels are continuing to improve, but I still need transfusions. Sometimes I go up to *Trèfle 3* to visit the nurses who looked after me.

Half vampire, half tourist full of new blood, I savour my wire-less illness. I'm taking strolls along hospital corridors, having showers and devoting myself to giving Rosy intense calf-rubs while she sleeps. I coddle my new life. I've got into a daily routine, incorporating seventeen drugs to be taken at precise times. My medicine bag is the size of a pillowcase. The pharmacists do nursing-lite. They bring me medicines at home to avoid me walking about among germs; they arrange to pick up my medication from a different pharmacy if they run out. They put their heart and soul into making my life easy. I sort my pills into Kinder Surprise capsules and drink enormous amounts of water to save my kidneys from the side effects of ciclosporin.

I down shots of St-Yorre mineral water and grenadine. Because of the corticosteroids, I'm on a no-salt, no-sugar diet. I keep getting the urge to demolish a jar of Nutella with a teaspoon.

I'm one month old and have the immune system of a baby. Soon, I'll need my vaccinations. I have to avoid anyone who's ill, anyone with a slight cold even. I have to put on my mask to go out. And still no public places. I'm in prison but at home this time, and my cell is indescribably comfy. Aftershave is forbidden, I can't even touch the packaging, but I gorge on Rosy's skin. She's oiling my brand-new gears with tender, passionate diligence.

I'm writing these few lines live from the egg chair, which I've just climbed back into. Stroking my scalp, semi-soft like an old tennis ball. I stem the flow of questions sweeping over me, so I have fewer answers to find. My best escape is still being creative. Invention. Teasing out the fragile and magical links between dreams and reality. Poetry is dessert for the mind, humour the cherry on top. And despite the cortisone, fruit is not off limits.

I'm learning how to sleep in my bed again. Flying in my duvet. What joy not to be woken up at 6am for a blood test, to tread the floorboards barefoot in the middle of the night. It's comforting to give yourself over to simple pleasures. Playing the ukulele, rereading my favourite books, pecking away at them chapter by chapter. Listening to records with a bowl of popcorn and watching films on the big screen in my room. A home cinema, until I'm able to go to a real one. Watching *The Return of the Jedi* for the tenth time and finding it even better than I remember. Savouring minuscule sensations with the epic appetite of a

Grand Canyon crossing. Letting the growing excitement over-whelm me: it's looking increasingly likely I'll get out of this.

My sister has come to see me. If I had stayed in hospital for two months, as planned, she would have been obliged to don mask, cap and gown. So her visit feels like Christmas dinner served early. We're warm and cosy, and for the first time in ages we don't have to pretend to reassure each other.

Shiver

2 December 2014

Today, I walked back to the hospital. I'd forgotten the looks you get in the outside world. It can feel aggressive when you're not used to it, particularly when you're wearing a mask. People look at me like a friendly monster, with varying degrees of politeness, obstinacy and gaucheness.

I crossed Place de la République at half speed, pleasantly surprised by the blinding sun. I frightened a little girl. Some people probably think I'm contagious. Others imagine the Elephant Man is hiding behind the mask. A few weeks ago it was nearly true.

I'm a survivor from an internal crash. My emotional taste buds are on maximum alert. Ordinary is extraordinary. In the depth of my bones, my new biological mother is making magical things palpable. Children dream of seeing flowers sprout from the ground before their very eyes. Like in a cartoon. Today, I'm witnessing such a miracle for real: my body is growing back! I saw myself dying, I see myself reborn. Soon, I'll be another me. Free to start all over again. The very thought crushes all sadness.

Redhead panache

24 December 2014

Downy plumage has started to sprout on my head. I'm going to buy shampoo for eggheads. I'm a chick hatching from his sterilized shell, gusts of wind buffet me this way and that, but I stay upright. Fingers gripping the sky, feet anchored on firm ground.

And so it goes around, the beauty of 'just maybe': I'm now free from transfusions! I can't take anything for granted, but I'm holding up. It means I'm not a vampire any more and I'm spending less and less time in pyjamas.

When I get my blood tests back, I can't believe they're mine. The results are too good for me. Body and mind have compensated so much for the lack of oxygen in the blood that now it's like I've got superpowers. When I was diagnosed I couldn't believe I'd become a vampire. Today, I'm just as blown away by the new hand I've been dealt. I'm back in the land of the living. Intact but fundamentally different. 'Oh me! . . . life exists and identity . . . the powerful play goes on, and you may contribute a verse,' proclaimed Walt Whitman. Oh passion! Oh patience!

Oh Dame Oclès, still mooching about in doubt's dark corners. The fact is, today I can live without other people's blood. I'm a haemato-poetic survivor. Everything is possible again!

I'm the oldest child in the world. And the youngest old man. A chimeric being with two mothers. Without the blood from the umbilical cord, Dame Oclès would surely have decapitated me by now. The professor told me the placental blood that is beginning to save my life comes from Düsseldorf. As my father was born on the German border, there's a considerable chance that a very distant branch of my family had a hand in this. My mother was Spanish but physically I take after the Lorraine side: freckles, pale skin and green eyes. Would I like to meet my new biological mother? I don't know. I think so. To thank her, more than anything. It's my turn to give *her* something. I'll have to scratch my head all the way down to the brain marrow to think of a gift as beautiful as the one she gave me.

For several months I'm going to be more fragile than a baby. A baby without an immune system, because the ciclosporin, which helps prevent my body from rejecting the transplant, will reduce the power of my own antibodies. But I'm heading for a return to an (extraordinarily) ordinary life. One giant baby-step at a time. Shimmering rays of hope are exploding all over the place. I look straight into the light rebounding off the mirror. I dream of new branches, I feel them growing, everything's trembling and vibrating anew. A bonus fifty years to *really* live. A fabulous firework finale. Now and always. My stubble's growing back, my hair's as soft as a baby fox's fur or a squirrel's tail. It's the return of redhead panache! I feel arrows of adrenaline coursing through my veins. They're turning into rockets. The countdown has begun, the emotional reactors are heating up and burning with pleasure. This time, I'm well and truly on my way.

'I am transforming, I am vibrating, I am glowing, I am flying, Look at me now,' sang Nick Cave. I have to get used to this idea: nothing will ever be the same again. Having my life saved is the most extraordinary adventure I've ever had.

Merci

On this journey into hell, I met various people who saved me. At death's door, I saw humans disappoint catastrophically. I saw others come into their own, become powerful and poetic.

Generators of hope, shiners of sweet light, with ceaseless refrains of think-nothing-of-it, you have saved my life. It all comes down to the details, to the accumulation of little things. I will never have enough new life to thank all those who supported me. Donors all – of love, of blood, of medical solutions and energy – you are my Walt Whitmans. Now it's my turn to try and be one too.

Thanks to Rosy, to Germain and Lisa, to my friends and family. Thanks to Professor Peffault de Latour, Lise Willems, the haematologist-with-the-kind-voice, Professor Didier Bouscary, Professor Gérard Socié, to all the staff of the haematological departments of Hôpital Cochin and Hôpital Saint-Louis, and to the pharmacists of Rue de la Bretagne.

Thanks to Olivia de Dieuleveult for accompanying me as I wrote this book.